"This book is an outstanding contribution to dementia care. Marguerite's experience, understanding, and compassion shine through every page. She has done a stunning job of presenting the complexities of dementia and how to be a care partner with the support of a mindfulness approach. Organized and inspiring, anyone dealing with dementia will be immensely grateful for this book, surely destined to become a classic in the field."

—**Olivia Ames Hoblitzelle**, author of *Ten Thousand Joys and Ten Thousand Sorrows*

"I highly recommend this exquisitely crafted, inspiring guide brimming with practical wisdom that flows from the depths of the author's authentic mindfulness practice and insightful dementia care-partnering experiences. The skillful dementia care principles seamlessly interwoven with mindfulness practices offer readers an opening in the heart and mind for extraordinary possibilities through the power of caring presence. This is a must-read for all who envision and feel called to actualize a 'radical new way for being more fully present for ourselves, as well as for the person with dementia.'"

—**Maribeth Gallagher, DNP, FAAN**, director of the dementia program at Hospice of the Valley in Scottsdale, AZ, mindfulness-based stress reduction (MBSR) practitioner and teacher, and mindfulness-based dementia care teacher

"With this clear and compelling guide to mindfulness practices, Marguerite Manteau-Rao fills an important void in the education of those who support people living with dementia. It is only by learning to be fully present that supportive partners can transcend com_____ cation barriers, understand distress, and creat_ ____ __ own well-being as well."

—**G. Allen Power, MD, FACP**, ___ *Beyond Drugs* and *Dementia Be*___

"Marguerite has designed a bridge for us to cross into a new era of understanding in dementia care where conscious caregiving and practices for cultivating awareness, compassion, and mindfulness are the new normal and standard of care. She beautifully illustrates the power of mindfulness practice to transmute caregiver confusion and dis-ease, which can be as challenging and debilitating as, if not more so than, dementia itself."

—**Laura E. Rice-Oeschger, LMSW**, coordinator of the
Dementia Wellness Initiative at Michigan Alzheimer's Disease
Center, University of Michigan Department of Neurology

"*Caring for a Loved One with Dementia* offers new hope that today's dementia caregiver can find a sense of peace in the difficult journey of dementia caregiving. Manteau-Rao does a masterful job introducing mindfulness, a practice that will be new to most caregivers. Her book provides real-world examples of where mindfulness can make an impact, as well as concrete suggestions for practicing mindfulness regularly. Caregivers who incorporate her lessons into their life will enjoy long-lasting benefits not just for themselves, but also for their care recipient."

—**Angela Taylor**, director of programs at Lewy Body
Dementia Association

"Marguerite has beautifully matched her own experience as a caregiver for a loved one with dementia with her mindfulness knowledge. The result is a book that meets the practical and emotional needs of family caregivers challenged by dementia. We dementia caregivers know all about stress, fatigue, grief, and sadness. This book opens us up to the possibility of moving beyond that by clearing our minds, opening our hearts, and partnering with our loved ones."

—**Robin Riddle**, CEO of Brain Support Network,
Parkinson's caregiver program facilitator at Stanford
University, and primary caregiver for her late father
with progressive supranuclear palsy

"Marguerite Manteau-Rao's mindfulness guide for caregivers helps outline the 'sweet spot' between the practice of mindfulness and caring for a loved one with dementia."

—**Elizabeth Edgerly, PhD**, chief program officer of the Alzheimer's Association, Northern California and Northern Nevada Chapter

"In this beautiful book, Marguerite applies her experience and compassion to gently guide a care partner as they learn to transform grief and loss into wisdom with loving-kindness. This book is the necessary platform for building a new perspective on changes we frequently face in the final phases of life. Each chapter provides another link in the lifeline that prevents drowning in our own thoughts and emotions."

—**Catherine Madison, MD**, medical director at Ray Dolby Brain Health Center in San Francisco, CA

"Marguerite Manteau-Rao has written an essential guide for caregivers supporting someone living with a dementia-related illness. A generous and skillful teacher, Marguerite shares practices that are beneficial and healing. *Caring for a Loved One with Dementia* is certain to help ease a seemingly impossible journey."

—**Roy Remer**, director of the Guest House and volunteer programs at Zen Hospice Project in San Francisco, CA, and teacher of mindfulness practices for professional and informal caregivers

Caring for a Loved One with Dementia

A MINDFULNESS-BASED GUIDE *for*
REDUCING STRESS *and* MAKING *the*
BEST *of* YOUR JOURNEY TOGETHER

Marguerite Manteau-Rao, LCSW

New Harbinger Publications, Inc.

Publisher's Note

"Informal Practice: Self-Compassion Break" is adapted from the work of Kristin Neff.

Distributed in Canada by Raincoast Books

Copyright © 2016 by Marguerite Manteau-Rao
New Harbinger Publications, Inc.
5674 Shattuck Avenue
Oakland, CA 94609
www.newharbinger.com

Cover design by Amy Shoup
Acquired by Melissa Valentine
Edited by Ken Knabb

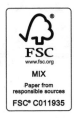

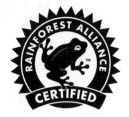

Library of Congress Cataloging-in-Publication Data

Names: Manteau-Rao, Marguerite, author.
Title: Caring for a loved one with dementia : a mindfulness-based guide for
  reducing stress and making the best of your journey together / Marguerite
  Manteau-Rao.
Description: Oakland, CA : New Harbinger Publications, Inc., 2016. | Includes
  bibliographical references.
Identifiers: LCCN 2015039308| ISBN 9781626251571 (paperback) | ISBN
  9781626251588 (pdf e-book) | ISBN 9781626251595 (epub)
Subjects: LCSH: Dementia--Patients--Care. | Dementia--Patients--Family
  relationships. | Caregivers. | Stress management. | BISAC: FAMILY &
  RELATIONSHIPS / Eldercare. | HEALTH & FITNESS / Diseases / Alzheimer's &
  Dementia. | BODY, MIND & SPIRIT / Meditation.
Classification: LCC RC521 .M365 2016 | DDC 616.8/3--dc23 LC record available at
  http://lccn.loc.gov/2015039308

Printed in the United States of America

18   17   16

10   9   8   7   6   5   4   3   2   1   First printing

To my mother, Mimi, whose journey through
Alzheimer's has inspired me to do this work.

Contents

Foreword

Mindfulness is a way of paying attention. It is a fundamental capacity of our human minds. In one sense it is completely ordinary, but what it can reveal is actually extraordinary. Using mindfulness, it is possible to awaken to the mysteries, challenges, and miracles of this existence. And I find it deeply reassuring that we humans can bring our full attention to something, whether it be difficult and painful or easy and pleasurable, and see it clearly, know it, and relate skillfully with it. There is hope with whatever we encounter in this human life.

Mindfulness is particularly well suited to this present time and place. It is a remedy for the speed of our lives in the modern world, the tremendous amount of distractions, the information overload, and the profound existential questions we face. As we rush around accomplishing so many things, traveling so quickly, communicating with so many people, taking in so much information, is it any wonder that we might crave a moment to stop, be in our physical bodies, attend to one thing fully, and allow our minds to rest?

Mindfulness is an ancient practice that has stood the test of time and has now spread throughout the world. Particularly noteworthy in the American journey of mindfulness is the development of the mindfulness-based stress reduction (MBSR) program by Jon Kabat-Zinn and his colleagues in 1979. This program was eminently successful and inspired a wide range of mindfulness programs that were adapted to specific populations: mindfulness-based cognitive therapy (MBCT) for people with recurrent depression, dialectical behavior therapy (DBT) for people with borderline personality disorder, mindfulness-based childbirth and parenting (MBCP) for pregnant women and their partners, mindfulness-based relapse prevention (MBRP) for people with addictions, mindfulness-based eating awareness therapy (MB-EAT) for people with eating disorders, acceptance and commitment therapy (ACT), mindfulness for people at the end of life, many different mindfulness programs for children and teens—and now, thanks to Marguerite Manteau-Rao, mindfulness-based dementia care (MBDC) for caregivers of people with dementia.

Just as mindfulness seems so well suited to our hectic modern American life, it also seems an exquisitely perfect fit for dementia care. The hallmark of dementia is that the past cannot be remembered. It is gone. Furthermore there is reduced capacity to think in (and plan for) the future. So the present moment is truly where the person with dementia dwells. What better way could there be to meet such persons than a practice that brings one's full attention into the present moment?

When I first met Marguerite, I saw her impressive gift for insight into the world of the person with dementia. This capacity for attunement I believe was born out of love for her mother, who had a long journey with dementia. We had this in common. My father has had Alzheimer's dementia for many years. Marguerite and I both had firsthand experience of the power of mindfulness to bring peace to ourselves and to those with dementia whom we loved. With mindfulness we both could see the full truth of our experience, and the truth was that there were moments of great tenderness as well as grief. My father became more emotionally transparent and we were able to easily express affection for each other for the first time in our lives. Even when he couldn't remember who I was, there were still such moments. ("You and I have been good friends for a long time, haven't we?")

In addition to her insight into the world of people with dementia, Marguerite brings her experience and skill as a social worker and psychotherapist into the design of MBDC. The program contains the humanity, compassion, and wisdom of someone who has traveled this road herself and accompanied many others. And finally, there is the key ingredient—mindfulness. Nonjudgmental, moment-to-moment awareness; this powerful, indeed extraordinary, capacity that we have to pay attention and be fully present for the richness of our lives. I am grateful to Marguerite for having written this book, which will help us all apply this capacity of mindfulness so that we can be present with those who have dementia as well as with ourselves. In these pages you will find simple, clear, wise help to bear the grief, find peace, and discover the full truth of the dementia experience.

—Kevin Barrows, MD
June 29, 2015
Founder and Director of Mindfulness
    Programs
Osher Center for Integrative Medicine
University of California, San Francisco
School of Medicine

Introduction

This book is for the millions of caregivers and family members who are caring for a loved one with dementia and who are looking for a better way to manage their journey. It is my hope that you will get a glimpse of what mindfulness—the practice of being aware of the present moment—can do for you, and how it can transform your interactions with the person with dementia. The mindfulness-based dementia care (MBDC) approach arose out of my own experience caring for my mother, who had Alzheimer's, and also from working with patients and families dealing with various forms of dementia. When the reality sank in about my mother, mindfulness became the one thing that helped me cope and make sense of her descent into dementia. Mindfulness also helped me better relate to her and even find joy in our shared moments. Working as a volunteer with Zen Hospice Project, I witnessed the same power of mindful presence as I helped care for the residents with dementia. Yet to my surprise, there was no mindfulness-based program specifically geared toward dementia caregivers. I set out to create one.

MBDC is a new, integrative approach that borrows from different perspectives in mindfulness, dementia care, and neuroscience. First is Jon Kabat-Zinn's mindfulness-based stress reduction (MBSR) program. Since its inception over thirty years ago, MBSR has paved the way for many other applications of mindfulness-based types of interventions with various populations, including now MBDC. Second is the Zen Hospice Project model of mindful and compassionate care for frail patients. From Zen Hospice Project I learned that mindfulness alone is not enough; it needs to be coupled with compassion and utter respect for the life ending process. Third is the person-centered care approach to dementia championed by G. Allen Power and other pioneers in the field. To Dr. Power I owe a deeper understanding of the interplay between the person in the caring role and the person on the receiving end. Fourth is the understanding of the dementia process through a neuroscience lens. The dementia field is still in its infancy, and much suffering arises from widespread misconstrued knowledge about the medical aspects of dementia. MBDC emphasizes neuroscience-based compassion. Fifth and last is a psychosocial perspective that embraces all aspects of the psychology of caregiving, including mental health for family members and caregivers. It has been very exciting to weave all these threads together into a coherent fabric upon which to rest the MBDC teachings.

In this book you will first learn about dementia basics, the different types of dementia, which professionals to turn to, and how to explore and understand symptoms. You will also learn about the connection between dementia care challenges and stress for you, and how mindfulness can help. Next, you will get a chance to become acquainted with some basic mindfulness practices that can become a part of your daily routine. I have purposely kept the practices very simple. My goal is for you to find at least one practice that works for you and that you can maintain. I am always amazed by how even just a little mindfulness practice can carry caregivers through and alleviate some of their stress. In chapter 3 we will explore how mindfulness practice can help you be with your grief while also attending to the grief of the person with dementia. Grief is an integral part of the dementia journey and it needs to be fully acknowledged. Mindfulness allows us to do the delicate dance of making room for the grief while not being overtaken by it. Chapter 4 focuses on the possibilities of enhancing the relationship with your loved one through mindful care partnering, a set of practices that blends stress reduction with compassionate care. In chapters 5, 6, and 7 you will learn how to make sensory awareness, heart practices, and mindfulness of thoughts parts of both your alone practice and your care interactions. Later chapters deal with how to integrate mindfulness into your communication and into your response to distress and challenging situations. We will also look into self-care and the many fruits to be reaped from this whole approach.

Developing the MBDC program has been a collaborative process. In particular, I want to acknowledge all those who have selflessly given of their time, energy, knowledge, and caring heart to make it what it is now. Bob Stahl, for teaching me how to teach MBSR and for his infectious passion for sharing the gift of mindfulness. Dr. Kevin Barrows, head of the Mindfulness Programs at UCSF Osher Center for Integrative Medicine, who provided the space, literally and figuratively, for MBDC to be incubated and take shape. Eric Poche and Roy Remer at Zen Hospice Project, who inspired me with the depth of their mindful care practice and teachings. Dr. G. Allen Power, who supported me in my early efforts to create a program like MBDC. Laura Rice-Oeschger and her team at the University of Michigan Alzheimer's Disease Center, who eagerly took on MBDC and nurtured it to make it an even better offering. Kathy Sniffen and Lori Wong, for helping shape MBDC during our community effort with caregivers in Modesto, California. Brooke Hollister and Leslie Ross at the UCSF School of Nursing Institute for Health and Aging, for advancing MBDC research. The Lakeside Park Specialized Elder Care community, including the clinical team, for all their support and commitment to the project. And last but not least, all the families, caregivers, and persons with dementia who have taught me so much about what they know and need, and whose ongoing feedback has helped fine-tune MBDC.

Note that throughout the book I alternate between the pronouns "he" and "she," since the information applies to either gender. Also, for the sake of brevity I often refer to the person with dementia whom you are caring for simply as "the person." At other times, however, I substitute the phrase "your loved one," as a reminder of your fundamental connection with this person whom you have been close to in the past and with whom you can continue to share precious experiences even now, regardless of what changes he or she may have gone through.

I hope this book inspires you to cultivate a mindful way through dementia care. You may start out simply wishing to find a better way to deal with the difficulties of caring for your loved one. But you may ultimately discover that the practice of mindfulness has much more to offer to you; it can open the door to a completely new life, a new way of being beyond just your role as a caregiver.

CHAPTER 1

Dementia Care, Stress, and Mindfulness

In this chapter you will learn about the connection between dementia care challenges, caregiver stress, and caregiver health. I will introduce you to mindfulness as the way to best deal with caregiver stress and to be the best caregiver you can be. You will also get an overview of the mindfulness-based dementia care approach that you will learn to practice in this book.

What Is Dementia?

When talking about dementia, it is important to understand the complex landscape of dementia. There is currently a lot of misinformation among both family caregivers and professional care providers. This lack of basic understanding is the source of much unnecessary suffering for both the person with dementia and the caregiver.

Not One But Many Dementias

First, you need to know that "dementia" is not one disease but rather an umbrella term that covers many different types of diseases, each with its own set of symptoms, causes, progression, and treatment. You should always question a dementia diagnosis that does not specify the type of dementia. At a minimum, it should recognize the need for further evaluation.

Domains affected by dementia include:

- Memory

- Executive functioning

- Language and speech

- Behavior and social skills

- Movement

- Visual spatial perception

It is useful to divide dementia-related diagnoses into three categories:

Neurodegenerative Dementias

These dementias are progressive and cannot be cured:

- Alzheimer's disease (AD) is the most common type and usually starts with progressive short-term memory loss accompanied by a noticeable impairment in daily functioning.

- Vascular dementia (VD) is caused by cerebrovascular factors, and often co-occurs with Alzheimer's, in which case a mixed dementia diagnosis is made.

- Lewy body dementias include Parkinson's disease with dementia (PDD) and dementia with Lewy bodies (DLB). Both of these dementias are characterized by motor symptoms and cognitive symptoms, including visual hallucinations. In PDD, motor symptoms appear first, whereas DLB starts with dementia.

- Frontotemporal dementias (FTD) include both behavioral variant types and language types. Memory loss is usually not a symptom of FTD, at least not until late in the disease.

- Less common types include progressive supranuclear palsy (PSP), corticobasal degeneration (CBD), Creutzfeldt-Jakob disease (CJD), Huntington's disease (HD), and posterior cortical atrophy (PCA).

- In about half of all cases, progressive dementias are mixed. This means that your loved one may have not just one, but two or three types of dementia.

Mild Cognitive Impairment (MCI)

While technically not a dementia, MCI is considered a precursor to Alzheimer's dementia. Similarly to AD, the first symptom is usually progressive memory loss. Unlike AD, however, MCI does not impact daily functioning. MCI does not necessarily lead to Alzheimer's, and memory-loss symptoms may remain stable for years or even improve.

Reversible Dementias

In these cases, dementia can be treated by taking care of the underlying causes:

- Cardiovascular factors: hypertension, cardiac disease, diabetes, smoking, stroke

- Metabolic abnormalities: hypothyroidism, hypoglycemia, sodium, calcium, heavy metals, or other compounds in the blood

- Nutritional deficiencies: thiamin (vitamin B-1), niacin (vitamin B-12), dehydration

- Medication side effects

- Psychiatric conditions: depression, anxiety, bipolar disorder, OCD, schizophrenia

- Injuries to the brain: inflammation, tumor, hematoma, seizure disorder, normal pressure hydrocephalus

- Infections: meningitis, encephalitis, syphilis, Lyme disease, HIV

- Delirium

Why You Need to Know

Knowing what type of dementia you are dealing with is essential for several reasons:

Treating Reversible Causes

For reversible dementias, it is critical to address the cause early on so as to prevent unnecessary physical and emotional distress from a misdiagnosis. Depression and delirium should always be ruled out. Addressing cardiovascular factors may help halt the progression of vascular dementia. And vitamin deficiencies should be treated to prevent irreparable damage to the brain. Normal pressure hydrocephalus can be reversed with a shunt in the brain to relieve the pressure from excess fluid.

Getting the Right Meds

What works for one dementia may be contraindicated for another type:

- Lewy body dementia responds adversely to typical antipsychotic, antianxiety, and anticholinergic drugs.

- Frontotemporal dementia responds adversely to cholinesterase inhibitors, benzodiazepine antianxiety agents, and typical antipsychotic drugs.

Because the field of dementia medications is constantly evolving, you need to stay up to date and go to trusted sources for your information. The websites for the UCSF Memory and Aging Center and the Mayo Clinic (see "Resources") are good places to start.

Understanding Distress and How to Respond

In the case of Alzheimer's or vascular dementia, the majority of behaviors are due to unmet needs. This is not true for frontotemporal dementia, in which behaviors are mostly internally driven. Similarly, visual hallucinations in Lewy body dementias are not a result of the care environment, but rather a manifestation of the disease itself. Armed with this knowledge, you will better know how to deal with challenging situations. We will discuss this in greater detail in chapter 9.

Connecting with Other Caregivers Going Through a Similar Journey

Tom, a caregiver, told me the story of joining a support group for Alzheimer's caregivers and finding himself unable to relate to others in the group. "Finally, my wife got diagnosed with frontotemporal dementia, behavioral variant, and I remember feeling so relieved at my first FTD caregiver support group. I felt I had found my flock. I could relate to everything those people were talking about." Every type of dementia comes with a unique set of challenges. Like Tom, you need to find the right flock for you—other caregivers dealing with the same type of dementia.

Planning for the Long Term

Different dementias have different prognoses. Knowing whether your relative has less than a year or more than ten years left will make a big difference in how you need to plan for the future. The progression of each dementia also varies, as do the symptoms and challenges. Armed with that knowledge, you will be better able to address financial, legal, family, work, housing, and care plan issues.

Participating in Clinical Trials

Knowing the particular dementia subtype gives your relative access to the latest treatment protocols, and possibly also a chance to participate in one or more of the many clinical trials taking place at any given time (see "Resources").

Who Can Help You?

I have found a great deal of confusion in caregivers' understanding of the different roles played by various professionals in the geriatric field. It is important to know what to expect from each one, whom to go to for what type of problem, and when.

Primary Care Providers

When you start noticing changes in a relative's behavior or functioning, a good place to start is a visit with your primary care doctor, family physician, geriatrician, or nurse practitioner. You will need to come in prepared with a detailed list of your observations, including a chronology of relevant symptoms, a medications list, a family history of dementia-related conditions, and the patient's medical, neurological, and psychiatric history. When listing the symptoms, keep in mind the six domains of functioning that may be affected by dementia, which I mentioned above (memory, executive functioning, language and speech, behavior and social skills, movement, and visual spatial perception). Also, as much as possible, make this consultation a partnership with your loved one.

Neurologist

If at all possible, try to consult with a neurologist as well. Besides performing medical and neurological exams, the neurologist may order additional tests, including lab tests, brain scans, and neuropsychological tests. Neurologists who specialize in dementia are called behavioral or geriatric neurologists and can be found in teaching hospitals or Alzheimer's Disease Research Centers (ADRCs). For a list, you can go to the National Institute on Aging website: http://www.nia.nih.gov/alzheimers/alzheimers-disease-research-centers.

Psychiatrist

Neurodegenerative dementias are neurologic illnesses, not psychiatric diseases. That said, dementia often coexists with, or can by be preceded by, psychiatric symptoms, particularly depression and anxiety. Dementia can also occur along with a long-standing psychiatric condition. When this is the case, it is important for neurologist and psychiatrist to collaborate on treatment.

Gerontologist, Geriatric Social Worker, or Geriatric Care Manager

None of these specialists are medical doctors. Their roles are mostly in the areas of advocacy, counseling, and care management.

The Extraordinary Stress of Dementia Care

Dementia tops other diseases in terms of the number and severity of the care challenges involved. This results in extraordinary stress for dementia caregivers, which in turn can lead to significant health problems. As a caregiver, you probably already know this firsthand, but it helps to realize that you are not alone.

Dementia Care Challenges

As you go down this list, think about your own challenges as a dementia caregiver. Does each item in the list resonate with you? Is there anything missing from the list?

- **Duration**
  Forty-three percent of caregivers of people with Alzheimer's and other dementias provide care for one to four years. Thirty-two percent of dementia caregivers provide care for over five years, and for some the journey can stretch as long as twenty years. Being a dementia caregiver is akin to running a marathon you did not sign up for (Alzheimer's Association 2015).

- **Multiple impairments**
  Dementia negatively impacts multiple aspects of functioning: cognitive, behavioral, language, and motor. This means

you need to care for the person not just cognitively, but also emotionally, socially, and physically.

- **Intensity**
  As the disease progresses, the person requires more and more care, to the point of complete assistance.

- **Unpredictability**
  During the early and middle stages of some types of dementia, behaviors and the ability to function can vary greatly from one moment to the next.

- **Lack of caregiver preparedness**
  Being an effective dementia caregiver requires a complete change of attitude and a sophisticated understanding of the person's needs. Traditional trainings do not adequately prepare caregivers for the ongoing challenge.

- **Practical challenges**
  The person's diminishing abilities present family members with financial, work, and legal challenges.

Dementia Caregiver Stress

The following statistics from the Alzheimer's Association 2015 Facts and Figures Report may help put your own stress in perspective:

- Fifty-nine percent of family caregivers of people with Alzheimer's and other dementias rated the emotional stress of caregiving as high or very high.

- Forty-seven percent of family caregivers report "a good amount" to "a great deal" of caregiving strain concerning financial issues.

- Forty percent of caregivers of people with dementia suffer from depression.

- Seventy-three percent of family caregivers of people with dementia somewhat agree or strongly agree that there is no "right or wrong" when families decide to place their family member in a nursing home.

- Fifty-nine percent of caregivers felt that, during the year before the person's death, they were "on duty" twenty-four hours a day.

- Seventy-two percent of family caregivers said they experienced relief when the person with dementia died.

Caregiving Stress and Your Health

I invite you to ponder the following questions as you consider the stress in your life:

Do you feel that because of the time you spend with your loved one you don't have enough time for yourself?

Do you feel torn between caregiving and trying to meet other responsibilities for your family or work?

Do you feel angry or strained when you are around the person?

Do you feel that caregiving affects your relationships with other family members or friends in a negative way?

Do you feel your health has suffered because of your involvement with your loved one?

Do you feel that you don't have as much privacy as you would like because of the person you're caring for, or that your social life has suffered?

Do you feel you have lost control of your life since your loved one's illness?

Do you feel uncertain about what to do about the person?

Do you feel you should be doing more for your loved one?

The chances are that you answered yes to at least some of those questions, possibly to many of them. Those yes answers can add up to a lot of stress! Although stress does not always translate into adverse health outcomes, the following information (Alzheimer's Association 2015) should give you reasons to pause:

- For some caregivers, the demands of caregiving may cause declines in their own health. Specifically, family caregivers of people with dementia may experience greater risk of chronic disease and mortality than those who are not caregivers.

- Forty-three percent of caregivers of people with Alzheimer's disease and other dementias reported that the physical impact of caregiving was high to very high.

- Seventy-five percent of caregivers of people with Alzheimer's disease and other dementias reported that they were "somewhat" to "very concerned" about maintaining their own health since they became caregivers.

Groundbreaking research at the University of California, San Francisco has also found scientific evidence linking chronic caregiving stress to premature cellular aging (Epel et al. 2004).

Why Mindfulness?

Jon Kabat-Zinn (1994, 4) defines mindfulness as "paying attention in a particular way: on purpose, in the present moment, and nonjudgmentally." If you are new to mindfulness, I would like to invite you to join me now in a simple practice:

Stay right where you are, and do not change a thing. Now close your eyes, and become aware of the sensations in your body, wherever they are most noticeable. Only do this for a few seconds. Then open your eyes.

You have just practiced mindfulness. What did you notice?

There are two main reasons why you ought to consider mindfulness practice if you are caring for someone with dementia: (1) to reduce your stress and (2) to help you be the best caregiver you can be.

Mindfulness to Reduce Your Stress

While very simple, mindfulness practice is one of the most powerful stress-reduction techniques at your disposal. Mindfulness is in fact a perfect antidote to the chronic stress-reaction cycle. Mindfulness mobilizes our parasympathetic system, the part of our autonomic nervous system that is responsible for rest, digestion, and energy conservation. By practicing mindfulness, we introduce the possibility of nonreactivity to external stimuli and we decrease the likelihood of self-induced internal stressors.

Over the last few years, neuroscientists have become increasingly interested in mindfulness. There are now numerous research studies that prove the benefits of mindfulness for our physical and mental health. Jon Kabat-Zinn's mindfulness-based stress reduction (MBSR) program has been the most studied. More than 120 experimental trials have shown MBSR and related mindfulness-based programs to have positive outcomes for various medical conditions, as well as mental health benefits, including stress reduction and improvements in anxiety and depression. MBSR is now widely used in hospitals and clinics. Mindfulness is also taught in schools, prisons, and workplaces. The "Mindful Revolution" even made the cover of *Time* magazine in February 2014!

I would like to make special mention of two research studies. The first one was a follow-up to the above-mentioned UCSF study on chronic caregiver stress and cellular aging (Epel et al. 2004). This newer study looked at the impact of mindfulness practice on cellular aging from stress and confirmed what caregivers who are practicing mindfulness already know subjectively: that mindfulness can help lessen their stress and restore a sense of physical and emotional well-being (Epel et al. 2009).

The other study worth sharing looked at the connection between mind-wandering and happiness. In this study, Harvard researchers Matthew Killingsworth and Daniel Gilbert proved the importance of keeping our mind on the present moment. Here is what they found (Killingsworth and Gilbert 2010):

- People's minds wander frequently.

- People are less happy when their minds wander than when they don't.

- This is true even when people are engaged in unpleasant activities.

Those findings have important implications for how to approach life as a dementia caregiver. No matter how unpleasant or challenging the moment, it is still better to be fully present for that moment. Your happiness depends on it.

Mindfulness to Help You Provide the Best Possible Care

Mindfulness can help you not just with stress reduction, but also with providing the best care possible. Here are some of the many ways in which practicing mindfulness uniquely equips you for care interactions with the person with dementia:

Calm, centered presence
With regular mindfulness practice, you will find that you are automatically more calm and centered, including during your care interactions. Calmness is one of the greatest gifts you can bring to the person in your care.

Not being limited by expectations or wishes
Mindfulness teaches us to stay in the present moment and to not let our mind wander in the past or the future. You will find yourself less likely to dwell in stressful mind states and more open to what each new moment brings.

"Being" versus task-driven

Many care challenges arise when we rush to perform a task with the person without first checking where that person is in that moment. Mindfulness helps us shift from a task-driven mode to a state of being with the other person. This results in the person feeling recognized and being more likely to respond positively.

Responding, not reacting

In the heat of a difficult interaction, we run the risk of reacting and making matters worse. Mindfulness practice trains us to take the time to pause before making an appropriate response. This way we are more likely to de-escalate tension and transform interactions for the better.

Awareness of the person

In our habitual rush to get things done, or out of habit, we may miss new cues about the person's mental and physical state. This is especially important whenever verbal communication is impaired. With mindfulness, you will be more capable of noticing nonverbal signals.

Awareness of environment

Mindfulness teaches us to be more aware of our environment, which also happens to be the environment of the person with dementia. In chapter 5 you will learn to use sensory awareness to better anticipate environmental stressors and to make appropriate changes in the person's environment.

Attunement

Mindfulness practice helps us become comfortable with dropping below our habitual mode of thinking and verbal communication. We learn different ways of connecting and signaling to the person that we are attuned to his or her present state. That skill becomes critical when the person with dementia is no longer able to speak or make sense when he or she talks.

Mindfulness-Based Dementia Care

The mindfulness-based dementia care (MBDC) approach takes full advantage of the potential of mindfulness practice to address the two main challenges for dementia caregivers: (1) chronic caregiving stress and (2) not knowing how to meet day-to-day care challenges. Thanks to the MBDC practices shared in this book, you will be able to transform the way you are with yourself and with the person in your care. In the process, you will be able to significantly reduce your stress and to reach a greater sense of self-efficacy in your caregiving role. You will also have the satisfaction of seeing your loved one respond positively to your new way of being in your shared interactions.

MBDC incorporates elements from mindfulness-based stress reduction (MBSR), the Zen Hospice Project approach to compassionate care, and an integrative approach to dementia that takes into account both biomedical and humanistic perspectives. Dementia care and mindfulness practice are interwoven throughout, so that in the end they become one and the same. The formal MBDC training program is typically spread over six to eight two-hour weekly sessions, with great emphasis placed on practice in between. Similarly, in this book you will be invited to practice in between chapters. You will get as much from the book as you choose to put in, in the form of your daily practice.

MBDC has been taught in a wide range of settings, including the UCSF Osher Center for Integrative Medicine, other academic institutions, adult day programs, assisted living communities, hospice organizations, and various community places.

A Positive Feedback Loop

MBDC enables you to initiate a positive feedback loop between you and the person in your care. This is in contrast to the all-too-common deterioration that may take place as a result of the chronic stress imposed by the dementia on both persons in the care dyad. It goes like this:

Caregiver's mindful and skillful presence

⇩

Initiation of positive experience with person with dementia

OR

Anticipation of not-yet-expressed unmet needs

OR

De-escalation of potentially distressing situation

⇩

Increased well-being for person with dementia

⇩

Fewer challenging interactions

⇩

Less stress for caregiver

Summary

- There are many types of dementias. Knowing which type you are dealing with informs treatment and care. If possible, seek evaluation from a neurologist with dementia training.

- Dementia care puts great stress on caregivers. Stress from caring for someone with dementia can be bad for your emotional and physical health.

- Mindfulness can help reduce your stress.

- Mindfulness can also help you meet your loved one where he or she is and provide the best care possible.

CHAPTER 2

Finding Out for Yourself: Practicing Mindfulness

Reading about mindfulness, we may gain a superficial understanding of the ways in which it can be applied in our lives. However, until we actually take the time to practice it, its benefits will keep on eluding us. In that sense, mindfulness is different from other dementia care approaches, with their more limited focus on "how-to" techniques. Mindfulness aims for something deeper, a radical new way of being more fully present for ourselves, as well as for the person with dementia. This attitudinal shift can only take place through steady, daily practice, the same way we may go to the gym every day to get our body in shape.

In this book, you will learn two different types of mindfulness practice. The first one, formal practice, is about setting aside time exclusively to cultivate the skill of mindfulness, and doing just that. The second type, informal practice, involves taking what you have learned during formal practice and applying it in daily life situations, including care interactions with your loved one. Formal and informal practices reinforce each other. Without the discipline of formal practice, it is unlikely that you will remember to apply mindfulness in your daily activities. And without ongoing mindfulness efforts throughout your day, it will be hard for the mind to settle enough to do formal practice.

Some Formal Mindfulness Practices to Start With

The following practices are typically taught to mindfulness beginners. They will constitute the base for your ongoing practice. They are simple, easy practices that anyone can do.

Only Five Minutes

Five minutes in the day—that's not very much. Five minutes: that's all it takes to give the mind a chance to settle a bit before the day starts. I first learned about the mindful check-in practice during my volunteer training at Zen Hospice Project. I can still hear Eric Poche's invitation to our group: "Let us sit!"

FORMAL PRACTICE:
Mindful Check-In

Choose a quiet place and a chair to sit in, and close your eyes. Then find your breath, wherever it is most noticeable in the body, and start to follow the breath. Whenever the mind wanders, as it most likely will, bring it back to the breath. Do this for about five to ten minutes. In the process, you will inevitably become aware of your overall state.

Other, fancier versions of the mindful check-in exist, but I am intentionally keeping it simple. If you can just remember to sit for a few minutes and pay attention to the breath, you will have made great strides in your mindfulness practice. I am always amazed at the diversity of the responses I get from caregivers doing this practice for the very first time:

- "My mind could not stop. It kept thinking thoughts."

- "This is the first time ever that I noticed my breath. I can't believe it."

- "Are you sure it was only five minutes? I feel so at peace!"

Resourcing with the Breath

The more time we spend with the breath, the more the mind gets a chance to settle and become calm. I recommend practicing awareness of breath for thirty minutes every day. At first you will benefit from the support of someone else guiding you. An audio file for this practice is available at http://www.newharbinger.com/31571; other files are listed in the "Resources" section at the end of the book. In general, there are a few guidelines to follow when doing this awareness of breath practice.

FORMAL PRACTICE:
Awareness of Breath

1. Paying Attention to Your Posture

First, make sure to take on a posture you can sustain easily for the whole thirty minutes. You can sit on a cushion on the floor cross-legged, the traditional way. Or, if you are like me and your body no longer allows you such flexibility, simply sit on a chair. Or if you cannot sit, take a lying-down position. You will just have to make sure not to fall asleep! If you are sitting on a chair, make sure to have an alert and at the same time relaxed posture. Imagine your spine lining up perfectly. That way your back will be less likely to tire. Also, make sure to uncross your legs and to have both feet resting on the floor. Then close your eyes. You are ready to practice!

2. Grounding Yourself in the Body

Begin by directing your attention to your feet, taking time to sense each foot resting on the floor. The feet—being farthest away from the head, where our thoughts take place—are a quick way to get us out of our ordinary thinking mode and into direct experiencing of the body in the present moment. We then continue with a brief scanning of the body at the different points of contact: thighs resting on the chair, hands touching or resting in our lap, buttocks and lower back against the back of the chair, ending with the middle and upper back; sensing the whole body sitting still, and along the way finding the breath where it is most noticeable in the body, then locking our attention on that place.

3. Setting the Right Intention

When practicing, it is important to set the right intention up front. In this case, all we want is to follow the breath as it comes in and out of the body. I tell myself to set aside any worries, plans, or thoughts for just those thirty minutes. This way, my mind can relax and I can proceed with the practice. I suggest that you do the same. Also, you may want to remember the benefits from practice. We do this to de-stress our mind, and it is one of the best things we can do for our mental and physical health. It is amazing how quickly we forget what got us to our chair!

4. Sitting Back and Watching the Breath

How we are with the breath can make a huge difference in the quality of our practice. Technically, "we" are not breathing. There is nothing volitional about the process of breathing. We only need to consider the fact that breathing continues during sleep while we are not even aware. The breath takes place all by itself; we need not do anything. During practice, we learn to find the breath wherever it is most felt in the body, then just sit back and watch the breath do its thing. We become aware of the sensations in the body with each in-and-out movement of the breath. That's all.

5. Keeping on Bringing the Mind Back

Of course, the mind cannot stay quiet for very long, and sooner or later we find ourselves wandering away. This is to be expected. We then just bring back our attention to the breath. We do this as often as necessary. Every moment of being with the breath is a time of being present and unified with the breath. It does not have to be pleasant. That is beside the point. When we lift weights at the gym, we may experience something similar. There is effort and pain involved, yet we keep going because we know it is good for us, it helps keep our body strong. Same here. The longer we can practice bringing back our awareness, over and over, to each breath, the stronger our mindfulness and the greater the benefit to be had.

6. Taking It One Breath at a Time

Last, I want to address the tendency of the mind to run away with impatience. Particularly if you are new to mindfulness, sitting for thirty minutes straight may seem like an impossible feat. I remember my first reaction when I arrived at a weeklong meditation retreat and saw the daily schedule posted on the outer wall of the meditation hall. Quickly, my mind computed: nine times forty-five minutes of sitting, plus six times thirty minutes of walking, made nine hours and forty-five minutes of meditation every day. Times six, it equaled fifty-eight and a half hours of doing nothing but sitting and walking, continuously, mindfully, for six full days. Of course, I was going to plough through, but still I noticed the aversion right away. Thankfully, the first morning the teacher gave an instruction for walking meditation that helped me view things in a very different light: "Only focus on one length (ten to twenty steps) at a time. Small intents are a lot easier than big chunks." Of course—one length, that I could manage. Even better, one step. Same with sitting meditation. We take it one breath at a time.

This awareness of breath practice is fundamental to mindfulness-based dementia care. It serves as a foundation for many of the mindful care practices that are a part of this method and that you will learn later in the book.

Getting into the Habit

Mindfulness practice involves taking on a new habit and sticking to it. Changing habits is never easy, and we need to take that into account when taking on this new practice. The last thing people who are already feeling overwhelmed by care demands need is one more thing on their to-do list. When introducing mindfulness to caregivers, I use BJ Fogg's "Tiny Habits" approach to behavior change.

"Tiny Habits"

BJ Fogg, a social scientist at Stanford University, believes that the tinier the habit, the easier it is to adopt (or to modify). New habits also need to be set up right. In fact, the trick is in designing such habits so that they are a source of positive emotions, leading to automatic behaviors. Tiny habits are things we can do at least once a day, in less than thirty seconds, and with little effort. Tiny habits must take place after a solid habit—or *anchor habit*—is already a part of our daily life. And we must learn to declare victory after each successful completion of a tiny habit. This is how we can rewire our brain to associate the new tiny habit with positive emotions.

The Sitting Habit

Here is how tiny habits can help you get started with your mindfulness practice.

1. **Pick a Place**
   Ideally a room that you can retreat to and where you will not be disturbed.

2. **Set Things Up Ahead of Time**
   A chair or cushion to sit on, and a streaming device from which to listen to practice audio files.

3. **Pick a Time**
   A time of the day when you can sit uninterrupted for thirty minutes is preferable. First thing in the morning is best, as the mind is still fresh and not yet encumbered with too much reactivity to outer events. This is also the best way to make sure to get your practice in. I have found it a challenge when I skip my morning practice to find the time later in the day. There seems to always be something else to do, and the practice keeps getting pushed aside. But if mornings are too rushed and the thought of getting up thirty minutes earlier is too much for you to bear, then, by all means, choose another time in the day that works better.

4. **Design the Tiny Habit**

   For the tiny habit, choose getting to the chair and sitting down for practice. The anchor habit can be getting dressed, or whatever activity you do first thing every morning.

5. **Practice the Habit**

   As soon as you are done with putting on your clothes, make a point of going straight to your meditation chair, and sit. At that point, you may start the audio file. Close your eyes and start listening to the practice instructions. Thirty seconds, that's all this process takes. Still sitting on the chair, congratulate yourself for having made the effort.

6. **Extend the Habit**

   Once on the chair, you will find that it is relatively easy to stay there and do the whole practice.

7. **Support the Habit**

   For extra help, particularly during the first few weeks when the new habit has not yet taken hold, share your progress with someone close to you who is supportive of your practice.

INFORMAL PRACTICE:
STOP

This simple, informal mindfulness practice, borrowed from mindfulness-based stress reduction, can go a very long way toward helping to decrease stress. It does not require any extra time from you and can easily be woven into your daily routine. For some dementia caregivers, STOP becomes a mainstay of their mindfulness practice.

At various times throughout the day:

1. Stop.

2. Take a breath, or more exactly find your breath and follow it coming and going in your body.

3. Observe the situation. What is the general atmosphere both inside and around you? You need not change anything; only be aware.

4. Proceed. Resume your activities.

The whole practice can be as short as one breath, or as long as you want. Visual reminders can be very helpful. Place a STOP sign in strategic places throughout your home or workplace: in the bathroom, by your desk, in the elevator, on the fridge, and so on. Another way to remind yourself to practice STOP is to attach it to a frequent daily habit. After all, STOP is just another "tiny habit" in need of an anchor. Here are some examples:

• Washing your hands

• Going to the bathroom

• Going through the door

• Opening the fridge

• Getting a glass of water

• Picking up the phone

How to Practice Mindfulness

How we approach our mindfulness practice matters more than any particular method we choose. Mindfulness is often misunderstood, and that's unfortunate. Such misconceptions can lead us to give up practice prematurely, or may prevent us from reaping the full benefits of true mindfulness. Hence the need to understand what mindfulness is and what it is not. Let's review some common misconceptions about mindfulness, as well as some helpful attitudes to bring to the practice.

Misconceptions About Mindfulness

Here are some common ideas about mindfulness that can get in the way of your practice, and some ways to change them.

"I Can't Stop My Thoughts"

Mindfulness is not about stopping oneself from thinking. Rather, it is about noticing when thoughts arise and then bringing the mind back to the intended object of our awareness (such as the breath). To expect the mind to not think is ludicrous. The brain is programmed to think, and we spend most of our waking life thinking. It is unreasonable to expect the brain to shut off its thinking mode just because we want it to. When we meditate, we realize we are not in control.

"A Few Minutes Is Good Enough"

Even mindfulness is not immune to our fast-everything culture. There are teachers and books that promulgate the idea that just a few minutes of mindfulness from time to time is enough. That is unfortunately not so. While it is true that a little bit of mindfulness is better than none, the reality is that mindfulness is just like any other skill. Practice a little and you will make little progress. Practice a lot and you will gain a lot. A good rule of thumb for mindfulness practice is thirty minutes of formal practice every day. I recommend first thing in the morning, as one is more likely to practice that way, and one can reap the benefit of one's early practice all day long.

"I Just Imagine I Am in a Meadow"

Guided imagery has its own set of healing properties, but it is not mindfulness practice. Mindfulness is about cultivating awareness of the present moment, not being taken away somewhere else. Next time you decide to meditate, remember to stay where you are!

"I Feel Worse When I Meditate"

With that statement comes the immediate implication that meditation is not a good thing and should be abandoned. This idea comes from the false assumption that mindfulness is about feeling good. While it is true that mindfulness often leads to feeling more peaceful and content within oneself, there are many moments along the way when practice may not be pleasant. It is not unusual for new meditators to feel physical and emotional pains they were not aware of before. Meditation is about being mindful of what is, no matter how pleasant or unpleasant.

"I Paint—That's My Meditation"

To get lost in the flow of a pleasurable or creative activity is not mindfulness, though it does entail the ability to concentrate, which is also part of mindfulness practice. When I used to paint for hours, I would get so absorbed in what I was doing that I would lose track of time. But I could not remember much of what had happened during all those hours. When we meditate, however, the opposite happens. The emphasis is on putting our full attention on the present moment and being aware. It also involves insight, the ability to learn about oneself in relationship to the present-moment experience.

Eight Attitudes

Here are eight foundational attitudes or qualities, adapted from Jon Kabat-Zinn's original list (1990, 33), that you will want to cultivate every time you sit down to practice mindfulness. Just read about them for now. As you practice, you will discover each one for yourself.

Nonjudging

Ideally we want to welcome equally every experience that comes our way. Of course, the untrained mind does not work that way. We are constantly evaluating ourselves and others. Knowing this, we make room for the judging mind, and our job becomes to acknowledge judgment as it arises and leave it at that. Maybe we feel anger arising at our situation, and we don't like holding that feeling in our heart. We need to be gentle with ourselves and recognize, yes, there is anger, right now...and then come back to our breath.

Patience

Mindfulness and impatience don't mix well. During practice, impatience can manifest in multiple ways. Maybe we want results, fast. We compare ourselves to others and wonder how come it is taking so long to get to the point where we can sit comfortably for thirty minutes or more. Or we want to rush to feeling bliss, and we don't want to go through unpleasant states. Or we can't sit still for "that long." We are used to doing, and to going from one thing to the next. Sitting still, doing nothing other than following the breath, requires that we temporarily give up our habit of impatience. We need to be patient with our impatience.

Beginner's Mind

Mindfulness is first and foremost about experiencing for ourselves each moment, without the filter of thoughts about how things ought to be. For instance, during the body scan, putting our attention on the left foot, the practice is about sensing what is actually happening in the foot. Maybe we find out there is no sensation there. The anticipating mind may rush to a conclusion and wonder, *How come? I should be feeling something in the foot.* The practice is to suspend that thought and instead be with the truth in that moment of "no sensation." All we know is that we never know what we might encounter from one moment to the next.

Trust

Practicing mindfulness, we learn to trust ourselves and our feelings. This is a gradual process. At first, we need to make room for the doubt and hesitancy that are likely to arise as we sit alone with our constantly changing experiences and with no one to guide us. It is helpful to remember that this is a practice. We need to allow for mistakes, and for not knowing. Eventually, as we deepen our awareness and our understanding, we will become more self-reliant and learn to trust not only ourselves but also the process of mindfulness.

Nonstriving

Practicing mindfulness, it is easy to bring in wishes and hopes for the practice. Maybe we want to be more calm, or we don't want to think, or we want to get rid of challenging states. Paradoxically, imposing goals on our practice is a sure way to prevent us from achieving those goals. When the mind busies itself thinking about what it wants, it can no longer focus on the present moment. While we need to put some effort into our practice, such as bringing the mind back to the breath, it is best to do so without any expectations of outcome. The best way to deal with striving during our practice is to recognize it when it happens—that's all. Then go back to the breath.

Acceptance

Acceptance means not pushing away anything that comes into our awareness. It starts as an intention and then gradually develops into a reality as we gain a greater understanding of the nature of mindfulness. We learn to accept and include whatever arises at each moment, including emotions, thoughts, and sensations that may not be pleasant or comfortable. At first, we may need to pay special attention to our resistance to such material. It helps to know that we all struggle with acceptance during practice. Our mind is wired that way. We also need to not confuse acceptance with condoning of undesirable material. Accepting the fact that we are holding hateful thoughts makes it possible for us to decide to not hang on to such thoughts, and to adopt loving thoughts instead.

Effort

Mindfulness practice takes effort. Left to its own devices, the mind naturally wanders, and when we start sitting we usually find out how challenging it is to keep on, even for a few minutes. It helps to remember the benefits of practice. The same way we exert energy at the gym to stay physically fit, we put effort into this practice to keep our mind in good health. At first we need to rely on others' accounts of the benefits of mindfulness. Eventually we will find out through our own experience. Continuing with the gym analogy, it helps to see the results from working out so hard every day. We become encouraged to continue, and the hard work becomes more tolerable. At some point, when the body gets in shape, we may even find some pleasure while exercising. When we practice mindfulness, the same thing happens. The more we practice, the easier it becomes. With effort also comes the pleasure of practice, even in the midst of difficulties or unpleasantness.

Self-Compassion

Heightened awareness needs to go hand in hand with self-compassion. As we are learning new practices, the temptation is to compare and judge how we have been doing things. Self-compassion entails being warm and understanding toward ourselves when we suffer, fail, or feel inadequate, rather than ignoring our pain or flagellating ourselves with self-criticism. Self-compassion involves recognizing that our suffering is part of the shared human experience, something that we all go through, rather than something that happens to "me" alone.

As you get further along with your practice, make a habit of revisiting the above list. You will discover that those qualities are all connected. You may resonate with certain ones and not others. In the end, each one will present itself to you.

INFORMAL PRACTICE:
Self-Compassion Break

Kristin Neff has a wonderful self-compassion practice that she freely shares on her website: http://www.self-compassion.org/exercise-2-self-compassion-break/. Here it is, adapted for the unique needs of dementia caregiving.

After you have spent some time sitting and practicing awareness of breath, put your attention on your heart. Notice what is there, the overall emotional climate. If and when you notice the presence of suffering, you may follow Kristin Neff's steps for a self-compassion break:

1. **Acknowledge the suffering.**
   Tell yourself, *There is suffering.*

2. **Acknowledge the universality of human suffering, particularly as it relates to being a dementia caregiver.**
   Caring for someone with dementia is a difficult journey. All other dementia caregivers are struggling just the same. "We are all in the same boat."

3. **Be kind to yourself.**
   What do you need to hear to help soothe your suffering? If you are suffering from depression, as many dementia caregivers do, that last step might be challenging. What would you tell another caregiver? Then tell yourself the same thing. Here are some examples:

   - *May I be kind to myself.*

   - *May I forgive myself.*

   - *I am doing the best I can.*

   - *This is a learning process.*

   - *No need to beat myself up.*

Once you have internalized the practice, you will be able to transfer it to situations in your daily life, times when caregiving interactions bring up challenging feelings and make you feel not so good about yourself. With time, you will learn to see self-compassion as an essential part of your mental health. Self-compassion is the first step toward feeling true compassion toward others, including your loved one, as we will discover later in chapter 6.

Setting Up Conditions for Practice

You can help by setting up conditions favorable to a daily practice. The main idea is to remove unnecessary hurdles while at the same time giving yourself as much support as you can. This includes having a daily routine that can fit within your existing routine and also not going at it alone. You will need guidance from a teacher and support from a community of practice.

Daily Routine

You want mindfulness to be as habitual as brushing your teeth every day. Do not wait. As the Buddhist teacher Ayya Khema (1987, 13) says, "If we didn't give the body a rest at night, it wouldn't function very long. Our mind needs a rest too, but this can't be had through sleeping. The only time the mind can have a real rest is when it stops thinking and starts only experiencing."

Start establishing a routine right away. Here are some tips:

- Practice every day.

- Focus on establishing the habit.

- Pick a time and place and stick to it.

- Start with a five-minute mindful check-in, then quickly increase your sitting time, practicing awareness of breath for fifteen minutes, then thirty minutes.

- At first, use audio files to guide you: http://www.newharbin ger.com/31571.

- Practice STOP often, using either visual reminders or anchor habits.

- Journal about successes and challenges with your practice.

- Remember why you practice!

A Teacher to Guide You

You can try practicing on your own. I will not discourage you! Using this book, you can definitely get started. However, in order for you to sustain your practice over the long run, you will need ongoing support from a teacher.

Fortunately, there are now more and more mindfulness teachers being trained, so accessibility should not be an issue. Technology is also making it possible to connect with teachers online when in-person contact is not an option. In the "Resources" section at the end of this book, I have listed several places for you to start if you are looking for a mindfulness teacher.

A Community to Support You

Without support from a community of practice, your practice is likely to wane, even with the best of intentions. The folks at Zen Hospice Project have known this for a long time with their mindful shift-change tradition. Volunteer caregivers at Zen Hospice start their shift with five to ten minutes of sitting together in silence, followed by a brief check-in, sharing where they are at that day.

Similarly, during mindfulness-based dementia care training, class participants are able to ramp up their practice quickly, in large part because of the support they get from practicing together over several weeks. Sitting in a group for thirty minutes of mindfulness practice makes it possible to overcome the mind's natural resistance to sitting still for so long. And in between weekly classes, students have the class experience to fall back on when they practice alone at home. Once the training is over, students are encouraged to find a community of practice to help keep their practice momentum going.

Ongoing mindfulness groups are becoming more and more common; they can be found in senior centers, hospitals, places of worship, and meditation centers. In the absence of any such group near you, you can always create your own. It only takes two people to form a group. During my trainings, I encourage people in the class to find a buddy, someone to call or text every day to remind each other about practice.

Summary

Teachings

- Mindfulness is a practice, not just something to read about.

- To help you get into the habit, start small and follow "tiny habits" principles.

- Cultivate the eight attitudes of mindfulness.

- Beware of misconceptions about mindfulness.

- Set up the right conditions for your daily practice.

- Find a teacher.

- Join a community of practice.

Practices

- Formal practice: Mindful check-in

- Formal practice: Awareness of breath

- Informal practice: STOP

- Informal practice: Self-compassion break

CHAPTER 3

Being with Grief

Grief is an omnipresent part of the dementia journey. It also represents one of the greatest challenges faced by both caregivers and
persons with dementia. Jacquelyn Frank (2008), a researcher at the
University of Indianapolis, asked 400 dementia caregivers the following question: "What would you say is the biggest barrier you have
faced as a caregiver?" Responses almost all centered around grief
and loss, and not the everyday practical challenges of caregiving. If
a similar study were undertaken with persons with dementia, it likely
would produce similar results. The only difference, particularly for
those further along in the disease process, would be their difficulty
in naming the deep grief they feel. Grief, whether in caregivers or
persons with dementia, cannot be ignored. It needs to be fully
acknowledged and reckoned with. In this chapter we look at ways
that mindfulness can help caregivers be with their grief throughout
the whole dementia journey. We also explore family relationships in
the context of dementia grief. And we delve into the grief experience for the person with dementia and what that means for caregivers intent on being there for their loved one.

Your Grief

Attending to your own grief as a dementia caregiver takes prece-
dence over anything else. It should not go unrecognized, or else you
run the risk of getting weighed down by powerful emotions such as

depression and anger. Dealing with your grief will help free up some energy that you can then use to take care of yourself and the person with dementia. I have found it helpful for caregivers to be able to put names on their experience, as well as to recognize the phases and different styles of the grieving process.

Three Types of Grief

Let us look at the three types of losses that make up dementia grief, and ways in which mindfulness can be used to effectively deal with each one.

Ambiguous Loss and Disenfranchised Grief

Pauline Boss describes the type of ambiguous loss faced by dementia caregivers as what happens when the person with dementia is physically present and at the same time psychologically absent (Boss 1999). Depending on the type of dementia, the psychological absence can be either cognitive or emotional, or a combination of both. With frontotemporal dementia, one of the hardest things for family caregivers can be the lack of emotional response from their loved ones. One caregiver, Betty, talked about feeling shaken after getting in a car accident and coming home to tell her husband, only to be met with complete indifference from him. With Alzheimer's, the loss is more of a cognitive nature, and spouses often talk about missing the ability to have an adult conversation the way they used to and having to be on their own for day-to-day tasks. With Lewy body dementia, the ambiguity of the loss is further compounded by the fluctuations in cognition that are one of the main features of that disease. The person may make perfect sense one moment but not the next one. The effect on the caregiver can be very destabilizing and can compound the sense of not knowing: Is my old husband there or not? Each type of dementia brings its own twist on ambiguous loss, but the one constant is the presence of that type of loss.

What makes ambiguous loss so challenging and difficult to acknowledge is the lack of validation from the outside world, particularly during the early stages of the illness. Your spouse may look just fine; he or she may even fool the doctor into an illusion of perfect mental health. But you know—you are living with your spouse every day and incidents become more and more frequent that leave no doubt in your mind. Trapped between the reality of your experience and this lack of external validation, you are left wondering and may be at risk of questioning the validity of your loss. You are suffering from disenfranchised grief.

Knowing about ambiguous loss and disenfranchised grief, and understanding that both are an integral part of the dementia journey, is usually a source of relief for family caregivers. Armed with that knowledge, you can then use your mindfulness practice to learn to recognize and be with your loss. Not trying to change anything, only allowing what arises in your heart, including the ambivalence, the confusion, and the not knowing. You practice doing this with great gentleness for yourself, realizing that ambivalence is one of the hardest emotional states to be in.

Anticipatory Grief

As discussed in chapter 1, knowing all you can about the dementia that is affecting your loved one is critical to effectively planning for the future. How many years is the person likely to live after the initial diagnosis? What are the stages of the disease? When should you expect drops in functioning, and in which areas? Answers to those questions can help you better prepare for what is to come.

That knowledge is also a double-edged sword. Your mind is likely to use that information to also start grieving the loss of your loved one's former selves long before those various parts of his or her personality and functioning have actually gone. That is how the mind is. The mind takes every bit of information and creates stories around it. And in this case, there is much material for the mind to run away with. The knowledge of what is to come, and our emotional reaction to it in the form of anticipatory grief, require that we bring our mindfulness practice into the picture, so that we do not burden ourselves with losses that have not yet happened.

Thanks to mindfulness practice, you will learn to catch your thoughts early enough, before they have a chance to create havoc in your heart. You will recognize when you are leaving the present and transporting yourself into a darker future. One way to deal with such thoughts is to say, "Not now," or a short phrase to that effect. You may also use the breath as a way to set your mind back onto the present moment. And as with ambiguous loss, you will do this with compassion for yourself, realizing that anticipatory grief is part of the course but that you do not need to let it take over your life. Mindfulness practice can also be used to make room for difficult feelings associated with anticipatory thoughts: feeling guilty for wishing away the person with dementia or for dismissing him or her prematurely as someone no longer able to contribute anything. Awareness represents the door out of the grief conundrum that is the result of the dementia disease process.

The Loss of Your Old Life

Dementia invites you to let go of your old life and to make room for a reality you did not ask for. This is hard, and demands that you grieve for every bit of your life before the illness. There is a method to this type of grief, starting with listing all your losses.

INQUIRY EXERCISE:
About Grief

1. Start by centering yourself with a mindful check-in.

2. Then, write down the list of all the losses you have experienced as a result of your loved one's dementia. You may use the following categories as a guide: dreams, hopes, roles, activities, relationships, finances, work, freedom, lifestyle, personal time, other. Write down whatever arises in the process, including thoughts, images, emotions, and physical sensations. There is no right or wrong. Trust your own process.

3. As always when dealing with grief, be gentle with yourself, and tenderly hold the thoughts and feelings that may arise.

Grief Milestones

Another way to look at this grief process is to consider the milestones in your dementia journey, usually significant events that marked a turning point in your life with the person. Here is a list of common milestones as reported by dementia caregivers:

- Person getting lost for the first time

- Phone call from your loved one's boss alerting you that not all is well

- Person causing a driving accident

- Hearing the diagnosis at the doctor's office

- Attending a caregiver support group for the first time

- Doing your first tax return on your own

- Your first time going on a vacation by yourself

- Your loved one's move to a residential care community

- Your first holiday celebration without the person

- Purchasing a wheelchair

- Sudden loss of speech due to a stroke

- The first time the person does not recognize you

- When the person no longer wants to eat

Are there any other events not on the list that have been significant for you?

Each time, use your mindfulness practice to recognize the sinking feeling in your heart, and become aware of the many ways in which this new loss is affecting you.

Next we will look at the different styles in which caregivers grieve, and what is needed for each style.

How Do You Grieve?

According to Kenneth Doka (2010), we tend to grieve in one of three ways:

Intuitive

Intuitive grievers "*feel*" their grief:

- They experience their grief as waves of emotions.

- They are overt in their expression of grief through feelings.

- They cope by taking time to grieve and sharing feelings with others.

- They run the risk of drowning in their emotions.

- They fit the common stereotype of grief as expression of intense emotions related to loss.

Mindfulness practice can help intuitive grievers be with their emotions, as discussed earlier in this chapter. It can also help them to avoid identifying with those powerful emotions. Caregivers might tell themselves: *This anger, this depression, this guilt are all part of the caregiving experience. I can make room for them, and let them pass. Meanwhile, I can go back to the breath as often as necessary, and I can continue to function.*

Instrumental

Instrumental grievers "*do*" their grief:

- They experience grief physically and intellectually.

- They are more discreet in the way they express their grief, and may appear as if they are not grieving.

- They show their grief by becoming hyperactive and immersing themselves in tasks and projects, including solving caregiving problems, memorializing what has been lost, and promoting causes related to dementia.

- They are reluctant to talk about their emotions.

Maladaptive, instrumental grieving for caregivers may translate into compulsive caregiving. Are you becoming overidentified with the caregiving role? Are you taking over and helping your loved one more than needed? Are you resisting help, or running yourself down? These are all signs that your grief energy has gone awry. Mindfulness practice can help you become aware of your overall state, and of the way your attitude and actions are having a negative impact on your health and on the well-being of the person in your care.

Blended

Most often, dementia caregivers combine both modes. You may find yourself going back and forth between "feeling" and "doing" your grief.

Mindful grieving makes room for those different styles. It also will enable you to go beyond any categorization and embrace your present-moment experience, whatever it may be. Part of your mindfulness practice includes letting go of any preconceived idea of what grief is supposed to look like, and of when and how it should manifest.

Learning from Zen Hospice

Zen Hospice Project has taught me quite a few things about grief, including the following list of principles. These principles are not just good for hospice volunteers. They can also help you hold your dementia grief in a mindful, loving way that will benefit both you and the person with dementia.

1. **Welcome everything; push away nothing.**
   With mindfulness, learn to be open to whatever the present brings, including pleasant and unpleasant moments.

2. **Bring your whole self to the experience.**
   We tend to think our way through life. Mindfulness is about shifting to a broader mode of experiencing, using all our senses. You learn to include physical sensations and emotions, as well as thoughts, in your awareness.

3. **Don't wait.**
   There is no moment other than this moment. The past is gone, and the future does not yet exist. Mindfulness calls you to live this moment fully. "Don't wait" is also an invitation to live each moment without regret.

4. **Find a place of rest in the middle of things.**
   With practice, you come to see mindfulness as a place of rest always available to you. In mindfulness, you can choose to unhinge from distressing thoughts and rest in each breath instead.

5. **Cultivate "don't know" mind.**
   Approach each moment with beginner's mind. Let go of ideas of how you are supposed to think and feel about your experience. Instead, make room for what is and the possibility of surprise.

All those precepts are interconnected. You may find that you resonate with one more than the others. You may also let them speak to you in your own words.

A Family Affair

For better or for worse, dementia grief is a family affair. Family members with close, loving ties may draw on each other for support. On the other hand, families with already weakened bonds may be unable to come together, or the dementia may become the source of added conflict. Dementia is the ultimate acid test of the marital and family unit. The good news is that you need not feel powerless in the face of family challenges.

Grieving Together

If you are fortunate enough to have at least one other family member with whom you can grieve, make a point of sharing each other's grief events and of acknowledging your feelings to each other. You may even want to create rituals that mark each step in your mutual grief process. That way, you will compensate for the risks of disenfranchised grief. If the outside world is oblivious to your grief, you can at least recognize it within your smaller circle.

Modeling Acceptance

Understanding the dementia grief process and the different ways in which it may manifest itself can help you be more accepting of other family members' reactions. You will be less likely to be annoyed by the "sentimentality" of your sister, who may be wearing her grief on her sleeve. Or conversely, you will not judge a parent who does not seem to care overtly or who may appear inappropriately cheerful. It will also be easier to deal with the grouchy relative who turns against you because of his grief-ridden anger. From family systems theory we know that change in one family member can impact the whole family. Resting on your mindfulness practice, you can start modeling a stance of openness, nonreactivity, self-acceptance, and compassion for the rest of your family members. You are doing this for yourself first, then your loved one, then the whole family.

Outside of the Family

It may happen that despite all your efforts, family members are simply not able to step into a supportive role, and the emotional cost to you becomes too high. You may need to psychologically remove yourself from the familial constellation and seek support elsewhere. Or it may be that it's just you and the person with dementia, and no other family members. Fortunately, you need not stay alone with your grief. You can find strength in sharing your feelings with others going through the same journey, preferably caregivers dealing with the same type of dementia. You can also seek help from a psycho-therapist familiar with dementia and caregiving issues.

Supporting the Person with Dementia

Not enough attention is paid to the grief process for the person with dementia. That grief is most acutely felt when people are conscious of their descent into dementia, and also during moments of occasional lucidity later on in the disease. It is present even when such people are aware of their condition only at a more felt, nonverbal level.

INQUIRY EXERCISE:
String of Losses

First, we need to grasp the extent of the losses from dementia, and their emotional impact on the person with dementia.

- Close your eyes and do a mindful check-in.

- Then, think of the person in your care. Go back to the first time you noticed a change in the person's behavior, memory, or ability to function. Write down all the losses experienced by the person since then. Some possible areas of loss to consider:

  - Memory

  - Language

  - Visual

  - Movement

  - Executive function

  - Activities of daily living

  - Professional

  - Hobbies

  - Sense of self

- Relationships

- Social activities

- Material things

- Home

- Driving

- Financial autonomy

- Legal rights

- Independence

- Purpose

- Self-esteem

It is not unusual for caregivers to come up with thirty, or fifty, or sometimes even more losses, each one significant on its own. The extent of the losses is truly staggering. Writing down such a list helps us empathize with the other person's grief. It may also give us a renewed appreciation for the resilience of the human spirit and our amazing ability to adapt, even with diminished cognitive abilities.

How Grief Manifests

There is nothing more heart-wrenching than witnessing a person's conscious loss of his abilities. Even far into the progression of dementia, it is not unusual for a person to have such insights. As one man put it, "I am losing my organization." This man had just moved into a memory care community and was looking for a way out, so that he could live the little time he still had left in the outside world "before I lose it completely." Another resident, who paced a lot, sat down and told me: "It is so difficult, the world I am in now. I am seeing myself slipping. My whole life, I went up"—she motioned with her hands—"and now it's all downhill from here." Metaphors are the way such persons let us into their grief. And when words fail, behaviors take over: pacing and repetitions to express anxiety and fear, agitation and aggression to let out anger, tears of great sadness, and apathy when depression and helplessness set in. One thing we can be sure of is the presence of grief all along.

Being with the Other One's Grief

As a dementia caregiver, you are left holding both your own grief and that of the person in your care. Being at ease with your own grief will give you the space to also be there for your loved one's grief. Here are some principles to guide you in your mindful companioning.

- **Seize the moment.**
  Grief does not have a set calendar. Ready yourself to set things aside whenever the person's grief manifests itself, whether verbally or emotionally.

- **Use your understanding of grief.**
  Always keep grief in the back of your mind, and learn to interpret what the person is trying to communicate.

- **Join in.**
  With both feet, join the person at her place of grief, and start exploring with her.

- **Stay in the metaphor.**
  Speak the same language, and relate through the person's metaphors.

- **Take the time.**
  Give the person the gift of your willingness to stay with her grief.

- **Provide comforting touch.**
  If welcome by the person, add a physical dimension to your intimate sharing around grief. Hold her hand or give her a hug.

- **Bring in the spiritual.**
  Give the person the spiritual comfort she needs. This may include reading religious scriptures or a favorite poem, or listening to a song.

- **Provide creative ways of expression.**
  Art making, storytelling, writing, dancing, and singing are some of the ways to facilitate creative expression of emotions, including grief.

- **End with remaining possibilities.**
  Always close by bringing back the person to remaining possibilities in the present moment.

- **Acknowledge the gift to yourself.**
  This is a mutual experience. Reflect on what you gained from this open sharing around grief.

The more you can be present for the person's grief, the less the need for the person to act out the distress of disenfranchised grief. Mindful companioning helps you get closer, not further apart, as you both grieve. Earlier in the disease, there may also be times when you both engage in a frank exchange around your respective experiences of losses from the dementia.

The Power to Choose

The more is taken away from us, the more we want to hang on. This is what happens to the person with dementia. Jane Verity, at her "Dementia Care Australia" website (2015), talks about the Five Core Emotional Needs that we all have, which can become a source of distress when they are not met. On her list is "the power to choose," which goes with the need to feel that we are in control over our own life. As a caregiver, there are two ways that you can help the person with dementia regain his power to choose. First, you can seize opportunities as they arise during your care interactions and invite him to be part of the decision-making process. The other way is to create opportunities specifically for that purpose. Either way, it does not matter how big the decision is. More important is giving him many opportunities to feel that he is in charge. Mindfulness practice can help you slow down and notice all the times when you can "ask." There is also such a thing as the art of enabling decision making for the person with dementia.

MINDFUL CARE PRACTICE:
Enabling Decision Making

Here are some guidelines for how to best enable decision making for the person with dementia.

- Because of the dementia, it is important to not overwhelm the person with too many choices. Two options is usually good.

- If you need to get some business done, frame the choices so that you can still proceed with the task at hand. Break down the task into small steps and check with the person at each step: "Which sweater do you want? The red one or the blue one?"

- Set the tone and start each interaction with one small, fail-proof decision—for instance, knocking on the door and asking if you can come in.

- If a task is involved, state the task, then immediately follow up with a choice: "Good morning, Mom! This is Kathy. It's time for you to get up. May I turn on the light?" And wait for an answer.

- Focus on present-moment decisions.

- Make up opportunities for your loved one to exert her own decision making.

Try it and notice how the person responds. How was the quality of your interaction? And how did you feel as a result?

"Sitting With"

Researchers at the University of Kansas Medical Center found that when doctors sat down during a hospital visit, they were perceived by patients as having spent 40 percent longer than they actually had (Gordon 2010). Also, patients had almost no negative comments about the doctors who sat down, compared to doctors who did not. The practice of taking the time to sit down with patients is not just good in hospital settings. It is also one of the core practices for caregiver volunteers at Zen Hospice Project, who are trained to "Sit, Breathe, and Listen" when tending to the dying. Here, we are taking this concept of mindful "sitting with" and enhancing it with a "power to choose" experience. It goes like this:

INFORMAL PRACTICE:
"Sitting With"

When the person is sitting or lying down, take the time to sit with the person first before asking her to do anything:

- "May I sit with you?"
- Wait for a response.
- Sit, breathe, and observe.
- Connect.
- Proceed with the task.

So simple and yet so powerful. "Sitting with" is an attunement practice that allows you to accomplish several things at once. First, by starting with a "power to choose" question, you immediately place the control in the hands of the person. Second, you signal to her your willingness to meet her at her level, both spatially and emotionally. "Sitting with" is also good for you. While "sitting with," you give yourself a chance to be present for yourself as well as for the other person.

Summary

Teachings

- Grief is an inherent part of the dementia journey.

- Dementia grief needs to be recognized and worked through, or else it can add to your stress.

- Knowing about ambiguous loss can help you avoid becoming disenfranchised from the grief associated with the many very real, yet unrecognized losses associated with dementia caregiving.

- Mindfulness can help you stay in the present and not add the extra burden of anticipatory grief.

- In caring for a person with dementia, you are also losing your old life, your dreams, and your expectations about the future. Those losses need to be grieved as well.

- If you find out about your own grieving style, you can use mindfulness to make it work for you.

- Family members can be a source of comfort during the long, drawn-out dementia grief process.

- Family members may grieve differently. This may be a source of conflict that can be moderated with mindful acceptance.

- Grief is also an important aspect of the person with dementia's experience.

- As a caregiver, you can be a mindful companion to the other person's grief.

- When people lose control, their need to be able to choose becomes heightened. As caregivers, we can help facilitate that need.

Practice

- Informal practice: "Sitting with"

CHAPTER 4

From Caregiver to Care Partnering

We may start as a child, a spouse, or a good friend caring for our loved one. With time, and as we become more and more absorbed into caregiving duties, a subtle shift occurs in which we become a "caregiver," someone whose identity becomes wrapped up into a defined way of relating to the person with dementia. We give care, and the other person is on the receiving end. This ends up being problematic for both giver and receiver. In this chapter we will explore ways to discover a more balanced approach to care that can be beneficial for both the caregiver and the person with dementia, and for their relationship. We will also add new practices to our mindfulness toolbox.

The Problem with "Caregiver"

When we identify as a "caregiver," we introduce an unnecessary rigidity into the role that we play with our loved one. This translates into us feeling burdened, overwhelmed, and also alienated from the person in our care. It is only a matter of time before we crumble under the weight of the enormous responsibility we have taken on. We burn out and we become depressed. We also run the risk of "positioning" the other person.

The Positioning Trap

Whenever we are faced with someone with a disability, one common response is to pigeonhole or "position" the person as less capable than he is. This kind of positioning is very common when we are confronted with persons with dementia. The work of G. Allen Power has brought to light this tendency we all have, and the need to acknowledge it when it happens.

What It Does

Positioning is exacerbated by visual cues such as, for instance, seeing a person slumped over and nonresponsive in a wheelchair. Positioning goes hand in hand with taking on a "caregiver" role, which implies a unilateral relationship without the possibility of the other person reciprocating. I witnessed the following exchange in a dementia care community: Margaret, a new resident, was being wheeled in a garden by a care partner. An activity person turned to Margaret's care partner and said, "It is sunny. Does she need a hat?" Margaret, not missing a beat, replied, "Don't ask her. Ask me. I know what I need better than her."

Note that the activity person was someone who is very much in tune with dementia psychology. Yet she got tricked by Margaret's appearance, and the natural tendency we all have to position elders with dementia. Many persons with dementia do not have Margaret's ability to verbalize their need. Instead, they are likely to react in one of two ways: either withdrawing and becoming walled in, or the opposite, getting angry and acting it out.

Explore: Repositioning

Thanks to mindfulness, we can catch ourselves as we get ready to interact with the person with dementia. You can go through the following steps in a matter of seconds:

Notice your thoughts and feelings.

- Do you feel pity?

- Do you think you need to do everything for the person?

- Do you assume the person does not understand you?

Use your awareness to reposition the person.

- Remind yourself of the person's hidden abilities.

- "There is a whole person there. He or she may surprise me."

Give the person a chance.

- Don't assume that the person cannot do something.

- Enable the possibility.

Care Partnering

Instead of getting stuck in a fixed "caregiver" role, we can shift our stance to care partnering, a more mutual and balanced way of being with our loved one. I was first introduced to this notion by G. Allen Power in his book *Dementia Beyond Drugs* (2010). Care partnering allows the person with dementia to take an active role in his care to the best of his abilities. It also frees the family member from carrying the whole load of the dementia. The possibility of a true dialogue between both partners is reintroduced, leading to less loneliness on both sides. We also learn to view the other person as our teacher about the illness and, in a way, as a constant invitation to practice mindfulness. You can still call yourself a caregiver since this is what most people understand, but what you do and how you are in relationship with your loved one is all about care partnering.

The Need to Be Useful

Another reason for you to engage in care partnering and to avoid the positioning trap has to do with the need for the person with dementia to feel needed and useful, which is also one of the Five Core Emotional Needs in Jane Verity's list. The need to be useful, along with the ability to make decisions, which we discussed in the previous chapter, are the two most important emotional needs you should consider when caring for your loved one. Over and over I have found that many dementia behaviors have their roots in one of these two needs not being honored. A big challenge for dementia care partners involves having to satisfy their loved one's need to feel relevant and useful, despite the person's shrinking abilities.

A Need That Does Not Disappear

We all need to feel useful and relevant. Our self-worth depends on our ability to contribute and to be recognized for our contributions, past and present. If we pay close attention, we can see the many ways in which the person with dementia attempts to satisfy that need:

- A woman at the nursing home asks if she can help clear the dishes.

- The husband picks up his briefcase and tries to get out of the house every day between 9:00 a.m. and 4:00 p.m., which is when he used to be at work before his dementia.

- The master horticulturist takes great pride in tending the garden at her assisted living place.

- He used to be an electrician and tries to "fix" the electrical outlets around the house.

- The surgeon thinks he is still working at the hospital and calls all his caregivers "nurses."

Mindfulness practice allows us to notice those cues and not dismiss them as unimportant. Another way that we can be sure to not forget is by letting ourselves imagine for a moment what it would be like if we all of a sudden lost many of the abilities that we take for granted. How might we feel if we could no longer hold our job, participate in chores around the house, or even help with our own care?

Shrinking Abilities

It's hard to continue to be an active contributor when cognitive abilities become compromised.

- The person can't remember what happened even a few minutes ago.

- The person can't initiate tasks.

- The person can't be trusted because of bad judgment.

- The person can't drive anymore.

- The person has trouble moving through space.

- The person can't verbalize what she wants.

- The person does not understand the meaning of words anymore.

- The person hallucinates.

- The person is okay one minute but not the next one.

- And many other difficulties that may vary with each type of dementia, and the stage of the disease.

Therein lies the challenge. The need to remain useful and to lead a meaningful life is still there, but the ability to fulfill that need is compromised. The person becomes dependent on her care partner to enable her.

How You Can Help

Answering the question "What can I do with him?" is not easy, but not impossible. Putting your head and heart into this quest will help you figure it out. In particular, I encourage you to complete the following inventory of the person's remaining abilities as well as a reflection on his life before dementia, and the types of roles that were important to him then.

EXPLORE:
Abilities Inventory

Think about the person in your care and make a list of activities, no matter how small, that the person can do on her own, or with some assistance. Use the following list as a guide and circle all the activities that apply:

Personal care:

- Waking up
- Picking clothes
- Getting dressed
- Toileting
- Shower/bath
- Brushing teeth
- Combing/styling hair
- Eating
- Drinking
- Getting ready for bed
- Walking
- Sitting

Work and hobbies:

- Professional job
- Singing
- Dancing
- Reading
- Writing
- Making art
- Playing music
- Playing games
- Others

Communication:

- Speaking
- Understanding

Chores:

- Grocery shopping
- Planning meals
- Assisting with preparing meals
- Setting table
- Cleaning table
- Passing out snacks
- Vacuuming
- Sweeping
- Folding laundry
- Sewing
- Sorting out things
- Feeding pet
- Flower arrangements
- Walking the dog
- Gardening
- Taking out garbage
- Recycling
- Fixing things
- Picking up mail
- Answering phone
- Others

- Caring for others
- Feeling emotions
- Expressing feelings
- Making others feel calm
- Helping with groups

Other abilities: _____

_____

Another way to think about abilities for the person with dementia involves doing a review of the different domains and seeing which abilities are preserved within each of the following six domains: memory, language, behavior, motor, visuospatial, executive. This latter approach is more based in neuroscience and may be more challenging for the layperson. You may want to ask your loved one's neurologist to assess the person's remaining abilities in each of those six areas.

EXPLORE:
Life Review

Lifelong habits do not go away with dementia. Instead, they continue to surface, begging to be satisfied, and it is our job as care partners to see how we can facilitate that process. This may require some creativity! But first we need to sit down and remember those habits. Very often care partners forget and do not make the connection between their loved one's behavior and old patterns. I once helped a wife put the two together after she complained about her husband's nightly requests to check on the car in the garage. After some probing, it turned out that her husband had been teaching night classes at the nearby college for over twenty years. Of course he wanted to make sure the car was ready to go! To help you review your loved one's previous roles and habits, I suggest that you take a pad of paper and start writing down every major role previously held by your loved one, including:

- Work, student, volunteer, hobby, community, and home roles.

- For each role: location, hours, other routines, travel if any, tasks involved, and relationships to other people.

EXPLORE:
Finding New Roles

You are now ready to tackle the next step of how to help your loved one feel more relevant and useful. Looking at the inventory of current abilities and past roles, and looking at your loved one's current behaviors, see what ideas come up for you. What role can you help fulfill that taps into the person's abilities? For instance, the woman whose husband was looking for the car every night was able to reassure him that he was all set to go to work, and that she would drop him off later. She was telling the truth. The adult day program had become his place of work, and they were all set for the next morning.

EXPLORE:
Reminiscing About Past Accomplishments

Sometimes all that is needed is to validate the person's past contributions, as in this experience of mine with Mr. Wang:

> *Every night, same story. A few spoons of pureed substance, a few sips of chocolate Ensure and Mr. Wang is done with dinner... "Did I eat enough? I want to go to my room." Efforts to feed him only result in more frustration. Mr. Wang cannot wait to sleep away his sadness.*
>
> *Body wasting away, down to a mere ninety pounds. Mind no longer to be trusted for remembering the simple things. Wife of sixty years at home and also wasting away, although in a different way. Family visiting, sometimes. The reality is Mr. Wang does not have much to live for anymore.*
>
> *Watching all signs of life seemingly withdraw in one such as Mr. Wang, a natural response is to believe what's being presented,*

and to not engage. This time is different. I ask him what kind of work he used to do, and am surprised to see him smile. "I have three titles, in engineering." It turns out Mr. Wang had a long career as a gifted engineer, after graduating from one of the best universities. He used to build bridges. As he tells his story, I notice Mr. Wang emptying his plate. First goes the mashed-up beef, then the zucchini, then the rice. He finishes up the chocolate pudding, and gulps down half of the Ensure. There is no more talk of him going back to his room. When one of the other residents starts entertaining us with a story, Mr. Wang breaks into a laugh. "She has a sense of humor." We joke about the woman's imperious personality. "She is my professor!"

Taking it up a notch, I ask if he would be willing to advise us on the "engineering" problems we have in the building. "Sure, I have three titles…"

We can revisit that place of pride as often as necessary. To us, it may feel repetitive and boring. For the person with dementia, it is medicine for his heart.

Care partnering makes sense all around. It can help transform our relationship to ourselves and to our loved one. And it is one of the big gifts we can offer the person with dementia. It is a shift from the traditional "caregiver" role we are used to, and we will need all the mindfulness we can muster to keep remembering.

Two More Mindfulness Practices

Now is the time to add more formal mindfulness practices to your toolbox. So far, you have learned how to be mindful of the breath and how to practice self-compassion. The next two practices have to do with the body. Learning to mind the body helps us move away from our habitual way of thinking toward direct experiencing of the present moment, which in turn helps us to be more attuned to the person in our care. The two new practices are mindful walking and the body scan.

1. Mindful Walking

Walking is a natural activity that is part of our everyday lives. Yet we pay very little attention to our steps. Here you will learn how to use each step, the same way you have been using the breath to stay present. Mindful walking is a very grounding and calming practice that can be especially helpful if you are feeling anxious or overwhelmed.

FORMAL PRACTICE:
Simple Mindful Walking

Choose a place where you can walk back and forth for fifteen to twenty feet, either indoors or outdoors.

- Slow down and pay attention to each step.

- Look ahead and slightly down.

- You may have your hands behind you or at your side.

- With each step, notice the sensations of the foot touching the floor.

- Whenever your mind wanders, acknowledge that and bring your mind back to your step.

- At the end of each stretch, pause and mindfully turn around.

- You may appreciate doing this practice with bare feet.

INFORMAL PRACTICE:
Mindful Walking in Daily Life

You can carry the mindful walking practice into your daily life. Any time you have the opportunity to walk slowly is a good time to practice. Once you get into the habit, you will learn to welcome such moments. Some caregivers have reported practicing while taking their dog out for a walk.

INFORMAL PRACTICE:
Mindful Walking With

"Mindful walking with" is another attunement practice that I developed as a result of my work with persons with dementia. Mindful walking with is similar to "mindful sitting with," which we examined in the previous chapter. This time, you combine mindful walking with mindful attention to the other person as she is moving through space with you.

- Let go of your own pace.

- Place yourself at the side of the other person, not ahead or behind.

- Ask whether she would like you to hold her hand.

- Pay attention to your own steps at the same time as you are modeling your pace after the other person.

- If you find yourself getting impatient or bored, notice the feeling, and then return to pacing with the other person.

- If the other person needs you to walk in front of her, adjust the practice accordingly.

If the person is in a wheelchair, you can attune to the person in a similar way:

- If you can, first kneel in front the person and make contact.

- Involve the person in the decision to move the wheelchair and go somewhere.

- Do not rush, and focus instead on the shared experience between you and the person.

- Be aware of the sensations at the point of contact between your hands and the wheelchair handles.

- If you find yourself getting impatient or bored, acknowledge this and place your focus back on the activity of pushing the wheelchair and the interaction with the person.

- Let the person know of any upcoming changes in pace, direction, or chair inclination.

- Once in a while, stop and make eye contact with the person, then resume.

It helps to remember that "mindful walking with" is both a stress-reduction method for you and a wonderful way to show the person that you are present for her.

---

2. Sweeping the Body

With the body scan, we go through our whole body, inch by inch, inside and outside. The object of our attention is no longer the breath, but instead each part of the body, one after the other. The body scan is a way for us to reconnect with the physical reality of our body, an aspect of our experience that is always anchored in the present moment. Every time we become aware of the body, we are being present. For some people it is easier to do the body scan than to be with the breath. The mind is more easily "entertained" for a long period of time, since it needs to keep moving from one part to the next.

FORMAL PRACTICE:
Body Scan

The body scan is best done at first with guidance from a mindfulness teacher. You may go to http://www.newharbinger.com/31571 for an audio file of the body scan. Rather than sharing the whole script for the body scan, I prefer to talk about the principles to take with you during the practice. That way you can make the body scan your own and keep on adding layers of complexity as you go along.

- You may practice either lying down or sitting on a chair.

- Close your eyes.

- Start with the left foot, then go up the left leg.

- Repeat on the right side.

- Scan the belly and lower back, then all around the waist.

- Move up to the front of the chest, then the back of the chest.

- Scan the left shoulder, front and back, then down the upper arm, all the way down to the fingertips.

- Repeat on the right side, starting with the right shoulder.

- Go to the whole neck, throat, face, and head.

- Pause long enough on each body part to explore all the sensations.

- You need not name the sensations, only feel them.

- If you cannot feel anything in a body part, be with the absence of sensations.

- Keep your emphasis on feeling the physical sensations.

- Notice any emotional reaction that may be attached to the part of the body that is being scanned.

- If your attention wanders to another part of the body, or to something else, bring it back to the body part under investigation.

- It can be tempting to fall asleep during the body scan if you are sleepy. If that is the case, do not lie down but practice sitting down instead.

- It is not unusual to feel nauseated the first few times you do the body scan. If that happens, do not be alarmed.

You can alternate between body scan and breath awareness practices. Just make sure to do one or the other every day for at least thirty minutes.

Benefits

When practicing the body scan, it is helpful to know and remember all the different ways in which this practice can be beneficial to us besides helping us stay present:

Releasing Tension

The body scan highlights the areas of our body where we hold tension, and with time we can learn to see the connection between our emotional reactions and our physical responses. Going through my stomach, I may find a knot and immediately get in touch with some frustration I did not know I was holding. Through mindfulness, I have the opportunity to give space for the tightness, both physical and emotional. Sometimes it is not so obvious and the body may be holding on to some old constriction. When that happens, we notice and let the sensation be without trying to think about an explanation. And then we move on to the next part of the body.

Managing Pain

Whenever we encounter pain in the body, we approach it differently from our ordinary way of thinking about "pain." Instead, during the body scan, we practice sensing all the physical sensations, whether pleasant or unpleasant, with equal interest and attention. And we tease apart the many sensations that make up what we are used to calling "pain": tingling, pulsing, numbness, hotness, coldness. We may give them names, or we may just sense them directly. More importantly, we get to see how we usually react to the painful sensation, adding an extra layer of unnecessary pain by tightening around it. Through mindfulness, we may give space for this reactive tightness to loosen.

Letting Go

Through the discipline of staying on one part of the body and then moving to the next, we practice letting go of whatever we could get attached to, whether pain or pleasantness. If we feel pain in our right foot, under normal circumstances our mind might want to go to that place, and it may be hard to think about anything else. With the body scan, we get to practice leaving our right foot and moving to the ankle, exploring the different sensations there.

Going to Sleep

Many times caregivers have reported to me that they use the body scan as a way to put themselves to sleep. The anxiety and depression often associated with caregiving can make it hard to fall asleep, or can cause one to wake up too early. Rather than lying in bed, tossing and turning, you can use that time to practice the body scan. Even if you don't end up falling asleep, at least you will have given yourself the gift of mindfulness and stress reduction.

Try these different practices and see which ones work for you. As you do, remember that mindfulness is not necessarily about feeling good while you practice. As long as you are able to follow the instructions and do the practice, you are doing well.

Wanna Breathe Together?

Can someone with dementia practice mindfulness? I get asked that question often, and the answer is yes, absolutely. The impetus for joint mindfulness practice often comes from the care partner having trouble finding time to practice alone. Inviting the person in her care to join her may be the only way she is able to do her daily practice. It doesn't hurt that mindfulness can also be beneficial to the person with dementia. Mindfulness practice can also be a simple yet powerful way for both to connect and engage with each other. Let us look first at the ways in which dementia impacts the person's ability to practice mindfulness.

1. Mindfulness and the Dementia Brain

Dementia presents both challenges and opportunities for mindfulness practice.

Challenges

Going over the various cognitive domains that may be affected, we keep in mind the following:

- Starting with memory and attention, the person's inability to hold on to new information, even for a short period of time, means we need to provide constant guidance and reminders about what it is we are doing, moment to moment, when practicing together.

- Compromised executive function requires that we jump-start the process and invite the person to join us, step by step, keeping our instructions very simple.

- When language comprehension is diminished, we can use touch and rely on the power of our mindful presence to inspire the person to follow us as we practice.

- When faced with impulsivity, compulsion, hallucinations, or other challenging behaviors, we need to lower our expectations and go into our invitation to mindfulness with a spirit of openness and flexibility. We may also want to choose our moment.

Opportunities

Paradoxically, dementia limitations also open the door to new possibilities for mindfulness practice:

- Because of memory loss, persons with dementia tend to be in the present moment, which is where we want to dwell when practicing mindfulness. Worries about the future and memories about the past no longer hold such a grip, and the mind becomes freer to simply rest in the now.

- When thinking becomes impaired, other cognitive processes take over. The person starts relying more on emotions, intuition, and sensory experiencing. That shift is favorable to mindfulness practice.

- Lack of self-consciousness leads to greater openness to trying new things, including mindfulness practice.

2. Implications for Practice

We learn to work within the limitations of the person, while at the same time taking full advantage of the opportunities presented by dementia. The following are some guiding principles and examples for you to keep in mind as you prepare to invite the person to practice with you.

EXPLORE:
Holding the Space

Of course, you will need to initiate practice. You will keep in mind the person's abilities, making sure to meet him at his level. Someone with mild cognitive impairment will be able to sustain a much longer practice than a person in an advanced stage of Alzheimer's. You can lead a practice yourself, or you can both listen to a recorded guided practice. Most important is to provide ongoing guidance so that the person does not get lost.

EXPLORE:
Choosing a Practice

Many types of practice can be adapted for the person with dementia:

- Breath awareness is a good place to start. Begin with a few breaths, then slowly increase the amount of time.

- Even simpler is the invitation to be silent together.

- A shortened version of the body scan can also work. You may focus on the feet and other points of contact. Or you can go through the whole body, only more quickly.

- A simple love practice involves asking the person to spend a few moments thinking about someone or a place she loves.

- You can direct the person to listen to pleasant sounds, maybe listening to a tape with waves or other nature sounds.

- You can practice mindful walking together.

All sitting practices can be done with eyes closed. If safety is a concern, you can hold the person's hand.

EXPLORE:
Going with the Flow

Practicing with a person with dementia demands that we provide some structure while at the same time adapting to the person's responses. You may even get ideas for practice you did not think of before. I would like to share a story that took place at an adult day program during the morning check-in with all participants and staff.

> We were sitting in a circle and I was guiding the group through some mindfulness of breath. At some point I was talking about the mind wandering, and how we bring it back to the breath. Jack, a boisterous participant, broke out of his silence with a very loud "I am thinking about my wallet." I used his sharing to reiterate my point about the mind wandering and how we bring it back. Jack responded again, this time with "I am STILL thinking about my wallet"—a perfect illustration of how the mind works. "That's right, our mind likes to persist in thinking about other things." Eventually Jack settled back into his breath.

Another time, Alicia, a woman with a habit of counting obsessively, was not able to keep silence with the rest of the group. I suggested that a care partner take her out for a walk instead and that they start counting their steps together. It was exciting to hear back about what happened after a few minutes of them going back and forth in the courtyard. Alicia was able to slow down and stop her counting. She became calm and relaxed, and the care partner got a chance to do her own mindful walking practice.

Including the person with dementia in your mindfulness practice can add another layer of richness to your interaction. And as we saw, dementia is not an impediment to mindfulness practice. It just requires that we adapt to the person's different way of functioning.

Summary

Teachings

- You can lighten your load by moving away from being a "caregiver" to care partnering with your loved one, turning your journey together into a team effort and not taking on all the burden.

- The need to be useful is one of the core emotional needs for the person with dementia.

- By being mindful of the positioning trap, you can learn to reposition your loved one as someone with many abilities still.

- Doing an inventory of the person's present abilities and reviewing his previous roles and routines can help you find roles for him.

- When present abilities are substantially diminished, reminiscing about past accomplishments can induce a sense of self-worth and purpose.

Practices

- Formal practice: Mindful walking alone

- Formal practice: Body scan

- Informal practice: Mindful walking with the person

- Exploring ways to practice with your loved one

CHAPTER 5

Coming to Your Senses

In this chapter we will look at the various ways in which the dementia brain responds to environmental stimuli and what that means in terms of care. We will examine sensory awareness practices that can help us become more attuned to potential environmental stressors for the person in our care, paying particular attention to sounds and mindfulness of hearing. We will see how sensory awareness can help us prevent or remediate various forms of sensory distress experiences for the person with dementia. And finally, we will explore mindful engagement opportunities around food, for ourselves and also involving the person in our care.

The Dementia Brain and Sensory Input

When exposed to sensory input, the normal brain is programmed to successfully process and integrate the stimuli. If I am in a loud restaurant having dinner with a friend, I will automatically tune out the surrounding noise and zero in on my friend's conversation. With dementia the brain loses its ability to effectively process sensory input. Placed in the same restaurant situation, a person with dementia will quickly become stressed and overwhelmed with the level and multiplicity of noises coming at her. As a result, she is likely to become extremely anxious and agitated. She cannot cope and she needs to leave the situation.

Let's take a closer look at the impact of sensory imbalance on people with dementia, and what can be done to remedy their distress.

Different Causes of Sensory Imbalance

Overstimulation

High levels of sensory stimulation create stress that the dementia brain is unable to process. Examples of overstimulation include:

- Bright lights
- Sounds (too loud, dissonant, or too many at once)
- Too much clutter
- Too many people
- Comings and goings
- Several senses stimulated at once
- Too many choices
- Not enough personal space
- Unwanted touch

The result is anxiety, agitation, and distress. Every afternoon, after a long day of busyness at the nursing home, Ruth loses it, and it does not take long before she yells, "Someone please get me out of here!"

Understimulation

Not enough sensory stimulation can be just as damaging to the person. We all need our senses stimulated. The consequences of prolonged sensory deprivation can be severe, even for someone without dementia. Sensory deprivation can happen in a number of ways:

- Not seeing familiar objects or people
- Lack of caring touch
- Food that is bland or not to the person's taste
- Lack of variety of sensory experiences
- Sameness in the days

- Lack of access to nature

- Not having a pet

- Lack of exposure to favorite music

- Monotone surroundings

- Being in a foreign environment

- Lack of pleasant smells

This can easily happen if the person is living alone at home and getting to the point of no longer being able to care for himself. It is also quite common in overcrowded nursing homes where there is simply not enough staff to engage in stimulating the residents appropriately. Common emotional responses to sensory deprivation include irritability, boredom, confusion, and depression.

Consequences of Sensory Imbalance

Sensory imbalance in the person with dementia often leads to distress that's expressed in various behaviors. We can read those behaviors as the person's best attempt to call for help and to stop an otherwise intolerable experience. When the sensory distress becomes prolonged, functioning may be impacted, sometimes permanently.

Common Behaviors

Behaviors in reaction to sensory imbalance usually fall into these three categories:

Stimuli Avoidance

Ruth means it when she demands to be taken out of her noisy floor. Her loud request is in fact totally appropriate given her level of distress, and the ignorance of the staff around her. Another resident might resort to another strategy, such as putting his hands on his ears to block the noise. Or he might ask to be taken to the bathroom, probably the only place in the whole building that is quiet at that time of the day.

Stimuli Seeking

In the absence of stimulation, the person will first attempt to seek what he needs. He may wander into other residents' rooms, looking for a change of scenery, new objects, or people. He may start asking for his family. Whenever she gets bored, Betty grabs her purse and starts "looking for a cab" to take her to her daughter's house.

Emotional Venting

When all else fails and the person feels stuck in her distress, anxiety and frustration can express themselves in a variety of ways, such as angry outbursts, pacing, hyperactivity, crying fits, or repetitions.

Functioning

Of greatest concern is the impact of chronic or acute sensory imbalance on the person's functioning. The person may become walled in or chronically depressed. In the case of delirium, this may happen suddenly, and as a family caregiver you should always be on the alert for any abrupt change in behavior, either extreme agitation or lack of responsiveness. Delirium is a common risk from hospitalization for persons with dementia.

Getting It Just Right

The responsibility falls on the care partner to provide just the right amount of sensory input, not too much but just enough, and the right kind. This can only be accomplished through a process of trial and error, based on careful observation of the person's responses to different environmental stimuli. In addition, exacerbating factors such as hearing and vision loss need to be addressed. Of course, we can only act on what we know. If we are not aware, we will not be able to address sensory imbalances ahead of time or we will not understand the cause of our loved one's distress. This is where sensory awareness comes into play.

Note: Helpful background for this section was provided by articles by Sophie Behrman and colleagues (2014), Lesley Collier (2014), and Heather Vasilopoulos (2010).

Sensory Awareness and Dementia Care

We as caregivers must "remember" to notice the various sensory stimuli that are coming at the person. This is made possible with sensory awareness practice, the practice of paying attention moment to moment with our different senses, with an emphasis on hearing, seeing, and touch. We practice sensory awareness first alone, by paying attention to sounds and other sensory input. Then we bring that same awareness into care situations, taking the information we glean from our sensory perception and using it to inform our responses.

Cultivating Sensory Awareness

Whichever sense we decide to focus on, the process is the same. We stop and intentionally put all our attention on using that one sense. Most commonly, we start with the sense of hearing.

FORMAL PRACTICE:
Mindfulness of Sounds

This practice can help reduce your stress, the same way as paying attention to your breath or practicing mindful walking. You can do this practice for only a few minutes or for longer if you wish.

- Sit and close your eyes.

- Put your attention on sounds.

- Notice how many sounds there are, and how loud they are.

- Are they coming from outside or from inside your body?

- Are the sounds pleasant or unpleasant?

- Whenever your mind gets called away, bring it back to listening to sounds.

INFORMAL PRACTICE:
Mindfulness of Sounds in Daily Life

You can bring the same mindful attention to sounds in care situations. Learn to pause often and simply listen to the sounds in your shared environment with the person in your care. Your formal practice is what will help you remember.

Caring with Our Senses

We bring all of our senses into caring situations, and learn to use the information gained in that way to improve the sensory experience for our loved one. Noticing potentially distressing stimuli, we make necessary changes in the environment, or we move the person away from the offensive input. Conversely, we take advantage of pleasurable sensory opportunities and share them amply with the person.

Sounds

Sound is at the top of the list in terms of its impact on persons with dementia. What do you hear? How might the present sound situation affect the person?

Too Much Noise

A loud noise, or too many sounds coming at once, can be too much for a person with dementia to handle. It is always a good idea to check with the person. ("It seems really noisy—what do you think?") The person is usually visibly relieved once the stressful noise source is removed. The earlier you notice the noise stress, the less likely the person will be to act on his distress.

Too Much Silence

Too much quiet time, too long, can be equally upsetting. Conversation, joining a familiar group, or sharing around the person's favorite music can be simple ways to break the dullness. Best is to combine pleasant sounds with social engagement with the person.

Seeing

Mindful seeing is about seeing what is really there, not what we *think* is there. Mindful seeing operates at several levels in dementia care situations.

Noticing Nonverbal Cues

Stop to notice what you see. How does the person look? What is his facial expression, posture, gestures? Does that tell you something about what he might need and may not be able to voice? A slight shiver may indicate that he is cold. Eyelids closing may be a sign of tiredness. We learn to listen with our eyes.

Seeing from the Standpoint of the Person

What does the person see from where she is standing or sitting? What might be disturbing? Or conversely, what might be a pleasurable experience? I once witnessed a woman trying to stand up from her wheelchair for no apparent reason. Only after I got close to her and sat by her side was I able to see and understand what was prompting her to move. The man eating across from her had snot dripping from his nose down onto his plate. She wanted to get a Kleenex for him!

Seeing with Understanding

Lastly, people with dementia can have trouble making sense of what they see and of the relationship between things in their environment. Do not assume they see things the same way as you do. The man bringing his empty cup to the doorknob is doing this for a reason. What does it look like once I let go of my judgment? The man is thirsty; he is trying to get water from what appears to him to be a faucet.

Touch

Mindful touch is one of the primary ways that we can continue to communicate our love and care throughout the course of dementia. Mindful touch can take over when words don't get through anymore. Though simple, mindful touch needs to be approached from several angles.

Knowing Ourselves

Before we can touch another person, we need to be aware of our own relationship to touch and to touching that person. It's better not to touch than to give a reluctant touch. If we are the hugging type, we need to be mindful of that as well, and keep in mind the possibility that a hug may not always be welcome.

Minding the Person's Comfort

When approaching persons with dementia, we become mindful of their relationship to touch and to being touched. With a loved one, we usually know, but even so, there is always the possibility that preferences may change as the disease progresses. We get a sense from watching the person's response to our touch.

The Gift of Holding

Persons with dementia, particularly in the later stages, often ask for their mothers. This yearning for the primal mother-child bond can be satisfied through firm holding of them. Sitting next to them, with one arm behind them and holding them tight, can make them feel safe again.

Allowing for a Different Experience

Mindfulness of touch is also about understanding what dementia does to a person's experience of the body being touched by other elements. For instance, the sensation of the water hitting a person's back during a shower might feel to her as though she is being beaten. Having her hair combed may feel painful. So we need to go slowly.

Spatial

Dementia may change people's perception of themselves in relationship to space, other objects, other persons, and even physical parts of themselves. Mindfulness teaches us not to project the way we think things ought to be based on our own experience. Instead, we make room for another reality, in this case the possibility of spatial challenges even in the simplest of daily activities.

People Approaching

Persons with dementia may feel threatened by someone getting too close to them, or coming from behind or from the side. Always approach from the front and slowly. Be aware of the space in between you and let them know your intention.

Sitting Down

For a person with dementia, being invited to sit down may feel scary, as if one might be going to drop through space. This applies to toileting as well. You need to be aware of the slightest inkling of fear, and reassure your loved one. You can hold both of the person's hands, for example, as you mirror lowering yourself down to an imaginary seat.

Holding Things

Finding one's hand's way to a glass of juice may not be that simple. An attractive colored plastic glass may make it easier to aim, and be less trouble in case of spills.

Temperature

Dementia can alter the perception of hot and cold. Hence we have to be extra mindful to not project our own preferences whenever temperature is involved.

Ambient Temperature

I remember once when a dementia patient complained of being cold and the aide refused to hear her. "It's not cold. I'm so hot," he said. The person with dementia may spend lots of time sitting and not moving very much. This makes it more likely that she will get cold, even when the ambient temperature is comfortable to everyone else. At other times the person may want to disrobe because she is feeling too hot, and we need to be sensitive to that as well.

Shower Temperature

Involve the person in testing the water with you before he steps in the shower. Also allow for the fact that water will feel colder on the whole body than when tested on the hand. There are so many subtle nuances that we need to pay attention to, on behalf of and with the person.

Food and Drink Temperature

A cold drink may make the person grimace, signaling that we need to warm it up a bit. The sensory system gets turned upside down with dementia, and we need to rely on the person to teach us what he needs, which is often not how we ourselves would like things.

Smell

One of our most basic senses, smell has a profound effect on the well-being of persons with dementia. Notice whether it is pleasant or unpleasant, and correct the environment so that the person is surrounded by pleasant smells, such as cookies baking, aromatic herbs, flowers, freshly laundered towels, and so on. Also, smell can be one of the ways that persons with dementia reconnect with past memories.

Caring with our senses is a practice that we can develop both "on the job," while caring for our loved one, and also alone, through formal sensory awareness practices. So far you have learned about mindfulness of sounds. Next, you get to add a few more practices to your sensory toolbox.

Three More Sensory Awareness Practices

FORMAL PRACTICE:
Walking with the Four Elements

This practice is a new twist on mindful walking, this time paying attention to each of nature's four elements: earth/solidity, wind/air, fire/temperature, and water/liquid. This is a great practice for when you are walking in nature.

- Starting with the earth element, focus on the solidity of the earth under you, and the solidity of your feet, and the contact between the two with each step. You are getting in touch with the solidity in you and around you. You can also observe all that is solid around you: trees, houses, cars, and so on.

- Next, turn your attention to the air element, starting with the breath coming in and out of you. Each breath is a manifestation of the air element passing through you. On a breezy day you can also feel the wind brushing against you. If you are inside, it may be feeling the fan on you. Get in touch with the air inside and outside.

- Next, shifting to the fire/temperature element, pay attention to the temperature outside and also your body temperature. Walking, you may notice subtle shifts in hot or cold places and how you react to those changes.

- The last element is the water element. There is water inside you, most immediately noticeable in the form of saliva in your mouth. On a rainy day it might also be outside you in the form of rain-drops or mist or drizzle. Near a stream or a fountain, you also get a chance to observe the water element.

- Once you have practiced with each of the elements, you can open your awareness to sensing whichever element is most prominent in your consciousness, moment to moment.

Walking like this in nature is a great mindfulness practice, with the advantage of not requiring any extra time in our busy days.

EXPLORE:
Raisins Exercise

I was first introduced to this practice by mindfulness teacher Jack Kornfield, many years ago. Raisins have never again felt the same. All you will need is one little raisin.

- Place the raisin in your hand and look at it carefully. Notice the difference between seeing with the assumptions of what a raisin is supposed to look like and looking at it as if for the first time. What do you see? Colors, shapes, surfaces?

- Next feel the texture of the raisin. Experiment with rolling it between your fingers or simply letting it rest on the palm of your hand. What are you finding out?

- Bring the raisin to your ear and move it around. What do you hear?

- Now bring the raisin to your nose and smell it. What do you notice?

- Next bring the raisin to your lips and notice how it feels. How is it to *not* eat the raisin yet?

- Place the raisin on your tongue and let it rest there. What do you notice? How does the inside of your mouth feel?

- Next, slowly chew the raisin. Become aware of all the steps involved and feel the actual taste of the raisin. Does it change during the chewing process?

- Last, swallow the raisin and observe the whole swallowing process.

What did you learn from this exercise?

INFORMAL PRACTICE:
Mindful Eating in Daily Life

Just as you did with the raisin, you can use mealtimes to practice sensory awareness and de-stress.

- Rather than rushing through your meal, take the time to taste and enjoy every bite.

- Do this in silence, if possible.

- Pause in between each bite, paying attention to your breath.

- Only eat until you feel satiated.

This practice is also good if you want to lose some weight. You will find you are less likely to eat more food than you really need.

During Meals

So much of life centers around food. This continues until the end of life. In fact, as dementia progresses and the field of possibilities narrows, food becomes even more important as an activity, a source of sensory pleasure, and an opportunity to engage with others.

More Than Just Food

Like Before

Dementia does not take away one's need to play prior roles. I have been struck repeatedly by the sameness of the responses from persons with dementia when asked to join for a meal by a visiting relative. Even late into the disease, the person will insist on wanting to host. "Can I take you out?" or more poignantly, "I don't have my wallet." As their loving one, we ought to help them save face. "Let me treat you this time. How about you pay next time?"

From Market to Table

Food is not just about eating; it's about getting involved in the whole chain of events culminating in every meal. This is what much of our home life centers around. That does not stop with dementia. We can try as much as possible to involve the person in the planning, harvesting, shopping, preparation, serving, and cleaning up for each meal. We can find ways to make the person feel useful to the best of his abilities. We can also look for ways for him to be involved in making decisions.

A Social Experience

As the dementia progresses, we may become tempted to serve the person separately from ourselves. This is especially true when we visit our loved one in assisted living. This is not natural and the person feels it acutely. "Aren't you going to eat?" He is looking for a mutual experience, where both you and he are eating together, preferably similar food. No one likes to be watched while he is eating.

INFORMAL PRACTICE:
"Eating With"

I got a call from a woman complaining about her husband eating too slowly. She gave me the idea for this "eating with" practice:

- Sitting, sharing a meal with your loved one, let go of your usual way of eating.

- Instead, become mindful of the other person's pace as she takes each bite.

- Use this opportunity to slow down and practice mindful eating.

- Model your pace after hers.

- Notice what happens in your eating experience, and the way you relate to the other person.

"Walking with," "eating with"—same thing. It is about shifting our stance from our ordinary, impatient, hurried way to welcoming the gift of slowness that is presented to us by our loved one, and using it to discover the benefits from shared mindfulness practice around the activity.

Assisting with Meals

People's need for assistance with their meals is bound to grow and change as their dementia progresses. From normal diet, to mechanical diet when food needs to be cut up, to pureed food, to pure liquid, to nothing at all, many transitions are to be anticipated. As care partners, we need to know when to make a switch. You will need to involve the doctor and to be especially careful of possible swallowing difficulties, particularly toward the end, but also for certain types of dementias.

EXPLORE:
Being Fed as a Grown-up

When the time comes, and our loved one becomes dependent on us for feeding, I know of no better preparation than to subject ourselves to the same thing. The following is a role-play I learned during my time with Zen Hospice Project. It will require you to practice with a friend.

- Have your friend feed you a meal.

- For interest, try to have a variety of textures—solid, soft, liquid.

- Make use of fork and spoon.

- Include drinking fluid as part of the exercise.

- Stay silent during the whole exercise.

- You can also try with your eyes closed.

- Notice how it feels to be totally dependent in that way.

- Notice the overall feeling, as well as your thoughts, emotions, and body sensations, throughout the experience.

What did you learn? How might that change how you assist your loved one with meals?

EXPLORE:
The Gift of a Delightful Meal

From Zen Hospice Project I also learned the art of mindfully tending to dependent ones with beautifully prepared and served meals. The fact that someone cannot eat solid food anymore, or that her mind cannot quite make sense of things, does not mean that she will not respond to tasty, tastefully displayed food. To the end, meals can be a feast for the senses and a source of delight for the heart. Here are some suggestions.

Make dining an experience that is both comfortable and pleasing to the senses.

- Offer meals at regular times, and in the same place.

- Talk to your doctor about the most appropriate consistency for the food.

- Pay attention to the presentation.

- Minimize noise and keep a calm atmosphere.

- Make sure the person is seated close enough to the table to reach for her food and drink.

- Serve in a mindful manner.

- Maybe put on some soft music.

- Check the ambient temperature and set it to the average comfort level.

- Serve comfort foods and drinks.

- Make sure the food temperature is just right—wait a bit if it's too hot, or reheat if it gets cold.

- Let the person eat with her hands if that works best for her.

Maximize choice opportunities, no matter how small.

- Facilitate; do not take over.

- Ask the person if she wants help.

- Give her time to eat on her own if she can, no matter how slowly.

- Lend strength to her by supporting her arm and hand as she brings food to her mouth (for the highly dependent person).

- Introduce choice at every step: when to eat, this food or that one, in which order, when to present the next spoonful.

- Offer food that maximizes the person's independence—finger food, or food that is easy to pick up with utensils.

- Do not overwhelm with too many food choices at once—one or two different items on the plate is good.

- Simplify utensils if necessary—offering only those needed for each course.

Engage the person.

- Sit down with the person.

- Position yourself so that you can make eye contact.

- Tell the person what is being served with each course, and the ingredients used.

- Match the person's pace.

- Make this a social event, including small talk and humor.

- Reminisce.

- Make this a mutual experience and share food together.

This practice is not just a gift for your loved one. It is also a mindfulness and compassion practice for you.

Summary

Teachings

- The dementia brain loses its ability to successfully process sensory input.

- Both overstimulation and understimulation can be stressful.

- Stress from sensory imbalance usually gets expressed through avoidant, seeking, or highly emotional behaviors.

- As care partners, we can best help by maintaining the most optimal sensory balance in the person's environment.

- But first we need to be attuned to our shared environment with the person.

- Sensory awareness can help us become aware of the sensory stress for the person when it happens—or even better, prevent it.

- Sensory awareness is also a stress-reduction practice for ourselves.

- Food and meals play an important role in our lives. Enjoyment from food becomes even more important in the presence of dementia.

- Mindful engagement around food is a lot more than just serving or feeding the person. It is also about engaging the person, and continuing to make the person a part of our daily life.

Practices

- Formal and informal practice: Mindfulness of sounds

- Informal practices: Mindfulness of other senses: seeing, touch, spatial awareness, temperature, smell

- Formal practice: Walking with the four elements

- Informal practice: Mindful eating

- Informal practice: "Mindful eating with"

- Informal practice: Mindful assistance with meals

CHAPTER 6

Tending the Heart

Caring for a loved one with dementia is a constant invitation to tend the heart. The garden metaphor is one that works well here. If we do not pay attention, the relentless demands from caregiving create the perfect conditions for negative emotions to take over our heart. These hindrances are like weeds. Left unchecked, they may obscure the possibility of love within. Fortunately, with mindfulness and its two sister practices of loving-kindness and compassion we can allow the possibility of love to flourish in our heart. Although this is not an easy task, it is necessary if we are to gracefully survive this journey with our loved one. All three practices are also linked to greater chances of better health for ourselves.

The Weeds in Our Heart

Those hindering mind states are all part of the human experience. They are the source of much of our mental suffering. We cannot avoid them, but we can use mindfulness to recognize them when they arise, and we can practice responding to them with wisdom and self-compassion.

Three Types of Weeds

Wanting What We Cannot Have

As a dementia caregiver, you may crave intimacy you can no longer have or the pleasure of an intellectual discussion that is no longer possible. You may want normalcy that is not to be had. You may want more time for yourself. So many things… With practice, you can learn to see how much extra suffering the mind generates whenever it wants something that is not possible.

Aversion to a Person, a Situation, or Oneself

Anger, rage, hate, depression, disgust, shame, guilt, and grief are all forms of aversion, either to internal or external factors. You don't like what is presented to you and you turn it into negative, dark, or fiery thoughts and emotions. Such aversive mind states are bound to arise in response to the many demands placed on you. You do, however, have the freedom to become aware of their effect on your physical and mental health. Unpleasantness may not be optional, but your aversion to it is.

Anxiety and Worries

When you find yourself worried, ask yourself, are the worries grounded in reality? Can you take some action to alleviate your fears? If not, the worries only add to your stress. In dementia care, it is only natural to give in to worries sometimes. You know the likely course of the disease, and it is easy for the mind to get ahead of itself and anticipate challenges that have not yet happened. Mindfulness practice can help you stay in the present and stop the train of anxious thoughts.

EXPLORE:
Mindful Inquiry into the Three Hindrances

The mindful way to deal with hindrances involves the following steps:

1. **Recognize the hindrance.**

   Ask yourself, *Am I suffering from wanting what I cannot have, or from aversion to the present situation, or from restlessness and fear?*

2. **Acknowledge its universal nature.**

   This is a hindrance. This is part of being human.

3. **Focus on the hindrance itself.**

   Rather than getting lost in the object of the hindrance, step back and become mindful of the hindrance itself.

4. **Acknowledge the suffering involved.**

   How does it feel in your body, your mind, your heart? There is usually suffering involved.

5. **Hold it with self-compassion.**

   Bring self-compassion into this mindful inquiry. In his "Transforming Anger" video Thich Nhat Hanh uses the lovely expression, "holding anger like a mother holding a baby." This is the invitation.

The weeds in the garden of our heart may not go away completely, but at least, through mindful attention, we can cut them short so that they don't take over. This opens the possibility for us to cultivate the love qualities that are most beneficial to us and that will help transform our relationship with the person in our care. The first such practice is loving-kindness.

Loving-Kindness

The practice of loving-kindness, or unconditional love, is not a mandate to feel love, but rather an invitation to explore our heart and see what happens when we extend a loving intention toward ourselves and others. Going back to the garden, imagine watering nascent blooms, every day watching them grow thanks to our careful tending. Eventually we may get to enjoy the delight from our garden, now full of beautiful flowers. This is what we can expect from practicing loving-kindness, over time.

Understanding Love

First, we need to understand what love is, and what it is not. Our common view of love is actually very narrow. We tend to only love based on certain conditions—that the persons we call our "loved ones" will behave in a certain way and will continue to give us the love we have learned to expect from them. Also, we tend to limit the field of possibilities, caring mostly about those close to us and not so much about strangers or those less likely to love us back. Dementia disrupts that way of thinking. Actually, the further along we are in the journey of dementia, the more forceful the call for us to embrace a more inclusive way of loving. The final veil gets drawn when the person no longer recognizes us. Our linear view of love ceases to be relevant and will only cause us more grief. Instead, it is better to learn to approach love on a moment-by-moment basis, with no expectations of being loved in return or of being remembered for our loving gestures. This radical shift has to take place in our heart if we are to move past paralyzing grief. It also happens to be one of the great secrets of a happy life.

Here is a poem I wrote about this kind of experience:

I visited once a very old woman.
I thought she was a man at first.
Age does that, obliterates all traces
of vanity and feminine glory.
A big, oozing wart on her cheek
kept drawing my gaze, hypnotic,
and in my heart, disgust surged.
She reached out for my hand.
Right next to my not-liking, love arose,
awakened by hers. She smiled.
"Have you had lunch?"
In her mind, I was her daughter.
I flashed back on my own mother
who had died two months ago.
And decided right there, why limit love?
I could become a daughter again,
if only for that moment.

Mindfulness and loving-kindness practice make it possible for us to notice and respond to what is presented to us with such insistence.

FORMAL PRACTICE:
Loving-Kindness

There are many ways of practicing loving-kindness. You can explore which one works best for you. Most important is the attitude you bring: open, curious, and making room for self-compassion. Here is how I like to teach loving-kindness to those new to the practice.

- Start with a mindful check-in, getting in touch with your body and the breath.

- Turn your attention to the heart and notice what is there. Are there any "weeds"? If so, try to hold them with compassion, using the self-compassion break you learned in chapter 2.

- You are now ready to do the actual loving-kindness practice.

- First, think of someone or something you love very much. It could be a small child, a pet, a parent, a lover. Whatever it may be, get in touch with the love and warmth in your heart as you think about that beloved being. Get in touch with the physical sensations in your body and the pleasant thoughts that arise. This is to help you connect with the possibility of love within.

- Now turn the attention to yourself and see if you can extend the same loving-kindness to the person that is you. If that proves difficult, as it often is, maybe you can visualize yourself as a child instead. Part of the practice involves saying to yourself words such as these:

  - *May I be at peace.*

  - *May I be at ease.*

  - *May I be happy.*

You can have as many phrases as you want. And you can make them your own. I have shortened mine to a simple *May I be at peace. May I be at ease.*

- Return to your most beloved image and get in touch with the warmth you feel in your heart. This is akin to resetting love to its highest setting. Send that tenderness and love to all the other persons in your life who are easy to love, whether alive or deceased—parents, family members, friends, teachers... Do this for each person, and each time repeat words such as these (or your own version):

  - *May you be at peace.*

  - *May you be at ease.*

  - *May you be happy.*

- Imagine how each person may receive your words. See the gladness in his or her face and get in touch with what happens in your heart. Is there happiness there as well, or do you encounter difficulties? If the latter, you can bring in self-compassion to soften the pain.

- Repeat with the following groups of people, in this order:

  - Neutral people, acquaintances, strangers

  - Difficult people, including those with whom you may be in conflict

  - Those experiencing physical or emotional pain or hardship

  - The person in your care

- Finally, extend the same loving-kindness to all living beings everywhere:

  - *May all beings be at peace.*

  - *May all beings be at ease.*

  - *May all beings be happy.*

- End with the breath.

FORMAL PRACTICE:
Opening the Heart Door

This practice arose out of my loving-kindness practice during the course of caring for my mother. I am happy to share it with you. It goes like this:

- Whenever you are thinking of someone, get in touch with your heart place and visualize the door of your heart. Is the door open or closed? How much love does it let out, or in?

- If the door is open, notice the sweetness of a fully open heart, and rejoice. If closed, even if just a little, notice the pain attached. How does it manifest in the body?

- What are some contributing thoughts? Angry, blaming, wishful, hateful—name them all, one by one. Thoughts about yourself, thoughts about the other person, thoughts about the situation.

- And then comes the hard part: Getting in touch with all the love in your heart, practice releasing those thoughts and visualize opening the door. See what happens, without judgment.

- If necessary, contemplate new thoughts, wise thoughts, to replace the old ones. And remember, it is up to you to open the door of your heart.

This practice can be useful when you are dealing with challenging relationships. This may apply to the person in your care. Maybe the two of you have a history and the disease is making it doubly hard, and you need to find a way within for an opening.

INFORMAL PRACTICE:
"Before Meeting"

Inspired by Olivia Ames Hoblitzelle's "doorway" story in her book *Ten Thousand Joys and Ten Thousand Sorrows* (2008), this simple mindfulness habit is a good way for you to de-stress while preparing to meet the person in your care. "Before meeting" is a combination of three practices you have already learned: awareness of breath, mindful walking, and loving-kindness.

- **Mindful walking**
  On your way to meet the person, walk slowly and pay attention to each step.

- **Awareness of breath**
  In between steps, be mindful of your breath.

- **Loving-kindness**
  Right before meeting the person, tell yourself the loving-kindness phrases you have learned, first for yourself, then for the person.

Compassion

Compassion goes hand in hand with loving-kindness. This time, instead of extending a loving intention, we get in touch with the suffering within the other person and we hold it with great gentleness. Compassion arises when we feel sorry *with*—not *for*—someone.

Four Steps

For dementia care partners, compassion can best be cultivated within the context of self-compassion, mindful attention, understanding of the disease, and last, skillful action.

Self-Compassion

Compassion can only take place after we have gotten in touch with our own suffering and held it with kind acceptance, as we have learned during self-compassion practice. We can only recognize and be with what we have already befriended within. Anger, frustration, helplessness, grief, sadness, boredom, outrage, shame, fear, and many other challenging emotions are part of our shared experience with the person with dementia.

Attention

In order to feel the other person's suffering, we need to pause long enough to notice his discomfort. Being too busy or overly focused on our own agenda are sure ways to sap any possibility of compassionate caring. Formal daily mindfulness practice is the best guarantee that we will naturally bring mindful attention to our care interactions.

Understanding

We need to be familiar with the symptoms and behaviors associated with the person's dementia. Only then can we make the connection between our felt sense of the person's suffering and the possible reasons behind their pain. For instance:

- If we know our loved one's dementia makes it hard for him to get his words out, we may feel compassion as opposed to jumping to impatience.

- Not remembering from one minute to the next has got to be terrifying.

- Being robbed of the ability to initiate any activity can make idle time feel stressful.

- Agitation can be due to the person seeing scary things that nobody else sees.

- Knowing our loved one is possessed by incontrollable urges helps us to not blame him.

This bringing together of the heart and mind makes it possible for us to take the next step.

Action

Compassion also has an active component. We feel the suffering and, if at all possible, we do something to help relieve it.

- First we meet the person in her reality, and we join her.

- Second, we lend her our mind without making her feel like a lesser person.

- We keep her safe, but not in such a way that she feels like a prisoner.

- We give her choices, but not too many, so she doesn't get overwhelmed.

- We help structure her days, so that she doesn't have to face too many blank moments.

- We don't mind the imaginary people that may be a part of her experience, but we seek medical help if her visions threaten her life or ours.

- We don't shame her for talking in ways that don't make sense to us.

And each time, we bring mindfulness to the effect of each of our good deeds on our well-being. Compassion, like self-compassion and loving-kindness, is beneficial not just to the person in our care, but also to our own mental and physical health.

How to Be Compassionate

Compassion is not that big of a deal. It is done without any expectations, and it does not need any big declaration.

No Expectations

Compassion is best expressed without any expectation of outcomes. We need to understand that being the most compassionate caregiver we can be is no guarantee that the person in our care will feel any better, or that the person will thank us. If we keep bringing expectations to our compassionate encounters, we run the risk of compassion fatigue. Through mindfulness, we can learn to pay attention to times when we start clinging to such ideas. Do you find yourself getting upset that your loved one's health is slipping? Dementia is hard that way.

Compassion Is Simple

One day, while sitting with Tim, a participant at an adult day center, I was struck by how compassion lies in the small things of everyday interactions.

He is one of my favorite people. Lewy body dementia has stripped him of many of his abilities. Eating has become a chore, and this morning I watch him struggle with breakfast. He has been served stewed peaches, cut up very small, a fried egg, and some oatmeal. Many times, I notice Tim attempt to pick up bits of fruit with his spoon. Each time, an empty spoon reaches his mouth. I offer to help. He lets me, but I can tell this is not easy for him. Eventually, he grabs the whole egg with his bare hand and eats it, just like that. It is clear that Tim has moved on to finger food. We need to listen to him, and no longer make him feel inadequate. The aide brings him a big slice of watermelon. Tim stares at the thing and does not touch it. How about cutting it into more manageable pieces? That does the trick. Tim finishes every bit of his watermelon and moves on with gusto to the buttered toast. A whole breakfast down, easy.

Thanks to mindfulness practice, we can learn to view dementia care as an ongoing experiment in compassion. We learn to notice what happens within ourselves when we feel moved to extend compassion to the other person—or the opposite, when our heart closes or our mind doesn't care and we ignore the call to lighten the other person's suffering. Eventually we become convinced of the goodness of compassion not just for the person in our care, but also for ourselves.

The Need to Love

We all need to be loved and cared for—that goes without saying. Less obvious is the enduring need we all have to care for others, even late into dementia. In most cases, dementia actually heightens one's ability to feel and express loving emotions. The heart takes over where the mind fails. I would like to share two stories to illustrate.

• Jane

She lives on the second floor, where folks are most challenged in their ability to communicate their needs. Jane also has a special friend, a small stuffed raccoon that she carries around. Yesterday, I stopped by and commented that this must be quite a special baby. "Yes, it is," she said, and caressed it with much feeling. Real babies and children long gone, husband dead, friends scattered in various homes, other residents lost in their own world—the opportunities for Jane to love are scarce. Still, the ever resourceful human spirit manages to get its needs met.

"You love him very much, don't you?" Jane turns to me and gazes at me deeply with her blue eyes and empathetically responds, "Yes, I do," and strokes her baby some more. Together we marvel at its sweet face. Does it have a name, I wonder? No, baby does not have a name, but Jane points to its glass eyes and black nose. She then puts it in its black pouch, and asks me if I want to hold it for a while. Feeling very touched to be entrusted with such a precious bundle, I thank her. "I love you," she tells me.

• "You Are Such a Good Mother"

My office is right on the dementia floor. I have become accustomed to Doris's loud, mostly incomprehensible monologue about "her baby." Doris spends a lot of time sitting by the dining room table, a familiar surrounding with her friendly aide always within earshot. Last night, I was about to leave when I caught Doris's inviting gaze. She wanted to connect. I came and kneeled by her side and mirrored her gaze. Nothing to do but be with her. Doris reached out to hold my face in her right hand. I could feel her care for me. In that moment, there was only a mother expressing her tender love for her child. "You are such a good mother," I said. Doris grabbed my hand, tight. I continued to let her love me. Doris broke our silence and asked, very clearly, "Are you all right?" Earlier that afternoon, I had had a disturbing phone call and was still dealing with the aftermath of one's unkind comments. Doris knew... I reassured her that yes, I was all right now. How kind of her to be so concerned. She really was such a good mother.

Once we understand how good it feels for the other person to love and care, we may create opportunities for such displays of affection. We also learn to seize such loving moments and express gratitude for the person's gift to us.

How Are You Doing with Your Mindfulness Practice?

Halfway through the book seems like a good time to check in on your practice. Although mindfulness can be a lifesaver for dementia care partners, it can be difficult finding the time and energy to take on and sustain the practice. Here are some common challenges encountered by caregivers who are new to mindfulness practice, and some things you can do about them.

1. **I don't have time. I am too busy.**

    - For the next few weeks, make practice a daily priority.

    - What can you take out of your day and replace with practice?

    - Make a point of practicing first thing in the morning.

    - Set your alarm clock thirty minutes earlier.

    - If you cannot find thirty minutes uninterrupted, break your practice into several smaller increments—five, ten, or fifteen minutes each.

2. **There is no quiet place for me to practice in my home.**

    - Make the best of what is available to you.

    - Include noises and other disruptions in your practice.

    - Use the breath or the object of your practice as a point of reference.

- Bring back your attention as often as needed, no matter how many times.

- Practice at times when your home is most likely to be quiet.

3. **I have trouble staying awake during practice.**

- This may mean you need to get more sleep.

- Pick times of the day when you are more likely to be awake.

- Avoid sleepy times such as after a meal or at the end of a long day.

- Do not practice lying down.

- Take a short walk beforehand.

4. **I can't stop thinking.**

- That's okay—your mind is just busy and needs time to settle down.

- Your practice is to notice what is happening—in this case, busy mind.

- Every time you notice the busyness, you are practicing.

- Every time you bring your attention to the breath, you are giving the mind a chance to settle.

5. **I am too anxious to sit for so long.**

- Include the restlessness and anxiety in your practice.

- Go back to the breath as often as necessary.

- Practice for shorter periods of time.

- If the feeling is too much, do a more active form of practice, such as mindful walking.

6. **I keep being interrupted by the person I'm caring for.**

   - See if you can get the person to sit with you, maybe holding his hand.

   - Practice while the person is asleep or engaged in a soothing activity, such as listening to music.

   - Find a place outside of home to practice—a church, the yoga room at your gym, in your car, at a friend's or neighbor's house.

7. **I can't do this. I am feeling discouraged.**

   - Appreciate the effort you have made so far.

   - Understand that new habits are hard to form.

   - Every day is another opportunity to start fresh.

   - Pick just one practice and do just that.

   - If you haven't done so yet, join a mindfulness community where you can practice with others.

Of course, recognizing those challenges goes hand in hand with appreciating all the efforts you have made so far. Maybe you have not found the time to sit faithfully every day for thirty minutes, but you have gotten into the habit of STOP throughout your days. Or you remember to be mindfully present as you sit or walk with the other person. Informal practice is an important part of mindfulness, and being dementia care partners presents us with many such opportunities.

Summary

Teachings

- Dementia begs us to open our heart to love.

- But first we must attend to the weeds in our heart, the three emotional states that are part of the human experience: wanting what we cannot have; aversion to things or people; and anxiety and worries.

- We can deal with these weeds through the three heart practices: mindfulness, loving-kindness, and compassion.

- The four steps to compassionate dementia care are self-compassion, attention, understanding, and action.

- Compassion without expectations attached is the key to preventing compassion fatigue.

- The need to love is universal, and does not change with dementia. Letting ourselves be loved by persons with dementia is a gift to them.

- Part of mindfulness practice is recognizing the challenges of practice along the way.

Practices

- Explore: Mindful inquiry into the hindrances

- Formal practice: Loving-kindness

- Formal practice: Opening the heart door

- Informal practice: "Before meeting"

- Informal practice: Compassion

CHAPTER 7

Clearing the Mind

Hopefully by now you have become more familiar with your mind, and the various ways in which it may trick you into unhappiness. Indeed, what we do with our thoughts is of the utmost importance for our well-being. Dementia caregiving presents us with many challenging situations, and each time we run the risk of reacting with unhealthy thoughts. This tendency gets further exacerbated in the presence of depression, a common risk of dementia caregiving. In this chapter, you will learn how to use mindfulness and wise understanding to clear your mind of such stress-inducing clutter. Mindfulness allows us to notice when our mind is getting polluted with self-pity, remorse, jealousy, or any number of other unhappiness-producing thoughts. Understanding allows us to know how to address the problem. Mind clearing is part of mindful self-care, along with mindful tending of the heart and other mindfulness practices you have already learned in previous chapters.

Are You Depressed?

Before going any further, we need to pause and broach the topic of depression. As we saw at the beginning of the book, caring for a loved one with dementia puts you at high risk for clinical depression, a serious mental illness that can cause you to see the world through a dark lens.

Finding Out

The most important step you can take is to assess the extent of your depression, and to recognize that unhappy thoughts do not necessarily reflect reality but may instead be a manifestation of the depression.

EXPLORE:
Depression Screen

This short depression screen (Spitzer, Williams, Kroenke et al. 1999) is commonly used by mental health professionals and doctors. I invite you to take it now. It will take only a few minutes of your time.

Over the last 2 weeks have you been bothered by any of the following problems? (Circle the correct number for each question.)	Not at all	Several days	More than half the days	Nearly every day
1. Little interest or pleasure in doing things	0	1	2	3
2. Feeling down, depressed, or hopeless	0	1	2	3
3. Trouble falling or staying asleep, or sleeping too much	0	1	2	3
4. Feeling tired or having little energy	0	1	2	3
5. Poor appetite or overeating	0	1	2	3
6. Feeling bad about yourself—or that you are a failure or have let yourself or your family down	0	1	2	3
7. Trouble concentrating on things, such as reading the newspaper or watching television	0	1	2	3
8. Moving or speaking so slowly that other people could have noticed; or the opposite—being so fidgety or restless that you have been moving around a lot more than usual	0	1	2	3
9. Thoughts that you would be better off dead or hurting yourself in some way	0	1	2	3

Add up your score and consider which action to take:

- Score 0–4: None to minimal depression. You need not take any action.

- Score 5–9: Mild depression. Watch carefully, and repeat the depression screen in a few weeks.

- Score 10–14: Moderate depression. Consider seeing a doctor and/or a counselor.

- Score 15–19: Moderately severe depression. Seek active treatment with medication and/or psychotherapy.

- Score 20–27: Severe depression. Seek immediate treatment with medication and psychotherapy if necessary.

Cognitive Distortions

Cognitive behavioral therapy (CBT) is a modality of choice to treat depression. It also happens to be very compatible with mindfulness practice. At the core of CBT is the recognition of the negative thinking patterns that contribute to our depressive mood. The first step is to recognize those thoughts when they happen and to identify the type of distorted thinking involved.

EXPLORE:
Inquiry into Personal Cognitive Distortions

Read the list below and identify which of these eleven patterns most apply to you (Burns 1989).

1. *All-or-Nothing Thinking:* You see everything in black and white. For instance, you get impatient with the person in your care, and you tell yourself, *I am doing a terrible job with him.*

2. *Overgeneralization:* You see a single negative event as a never-ending pattern of defeat, and you use extreme words such as "always" or "never." For instance, you are having a difficult

morning with your loved one, and you think, *I am tired of him always acting out.*

3. *Mental Filter:* You filter your experiences so that you only retain negative elements. For example, you were short once with your husband after he repeated himself many times, and all you can think about are the words you used that one day.

4. *Disqualifying the Positive:* You reject positive experiences and insist they don't count. For instance, your friends tell you what a devoted wife you are. Your immediate thought is *They are just saying that to be nice.*

5. *Mind Reading:* You assume someone's reaction is negative toward you, without really knowing. For example, someone in your support group fails to acknowledge you when you arrive, and you think she must be upset with you. *What did I do wrong?* During the group discussion, you find out her husband has been hospitalized and she is very distressed.

6. *Fortune Teller Error:* You anticipate that things will turn out badly, and you treat your prediction as a fact. For example, upon learning about your loved one's dementia diagnosis, you anticipate that your life is going to be miserable and you tell yourself, *It's going to be all downhill from here.*

7. *Magnification (Catastrophizing) or Minimization:* When comparing yourself to others, you always come up short. For instance, you may compare yourself to others in your support group and think, *They are so good with their loved ones, unlike me.*

8. *Emotional Reasoning:* You think your negative emotions reflect the way things are. For example, you think, *I feel useless, therefore I am useless.*

9. *Labeling and Mislabeling:* When someone else's behavior rubs you the wrong way, you attach a negative label to that person. Your husband with dementia is acting strangely and you think to yourself, *He's demented*, as opposed to *He has dementia.* Similarly, instead of seeing yourself as someone who is struggling to find patience, you tell yourself, *I'm a lousy caregiver.*

10. *Personalization:* You take responsibility for some negative external event when in fact you don't have anything to do with it. For example, your loved one is crying inconsolably and you immediately find yourself responsible for her sadness. *I must have done something to cause her such despair.*

11. *"Should" Statements:* You make excessive use of "should" and "shouldn't," and also of "must" and "ought." These statements set you up for feeling guilty, resentful, and pressured. When directed toward others, "should" statements are likely to cause you to feel anger, frustration, and resentment. For instance, you tell yourself you *should* always be patient with your loved one.

By simply labeling those thoughts, we are able to distance ourselves from them and let go of them more easily. We can also make the connection between such thoughts and our mood. Eventually we can start to recognize the patterns that tend to govern our lives. Mindfulness practice will allow you to notice the thoughts as they occur. One tendency to guard against, when learning to recognize cognitive distortions, is to avoid going to a place of self-blame for harboring such thoughts. I find it helpful to remind people that these are tendencies we all have, just like difficult emotional states. It is important to hold these thoughts with compassion and forgiveness for ourselves.

If you want to find out more about CBT, I invite you to explore the many excellent resources available either online or in books. You can also search for a therapist specializing in CBT, or even better, mindfulness-based cognitive therapy (MBCT).

Preventing Getting Depressed

Depression usually does not happen all at once, but instead creeps in slowly. There is a lot you can do to prevent it from taking over your life. It may still not be enough to ward it off, but at least you will have taken care of yourself in the best way that you can.

Share with Someone Who Cares: Depression Warning Signs

Given that you are at risk, it helps to have a good friend or a close family member watch out for warning signs:

- You are not behaving like your old self.

- You are not returning phone calls.

- You stay home a lot.

- You are dropping out of your regular activities.

- Your are becoming irritable.

- Your thoughts are more negative.

- You are gaining or losing weight.

- You are not able to sleep.

Make a pact with your friend that she is to let you know when she notices you going down, and that you will seek help if that happens.

Six Ways to Prevent Depression

To put all the odds on your side, you can also adopt a depression-proof lifestyle:

- Get enough sleep, exercise, and eat well.

- Socialize; do not isolate yourself.

- Force yourself to be active, even if you don't feel like it.

- Put some structure into your days.

- Recognize negative thoughts and try to cultivate healthier thoughts instead.

- Be on the lookout for warning signs and get professional help early.

The longer you let the depression take hold of you, the more challenging it will be to get out of it. Hence the importance of catching it early if you can.

Last, for those of you who have experienced prior bouts of depression, or for whom depression has been a lifelong struggle, the challenge may be in learning how to live with the depression. Mindfulness practice can become one of your greatest assets because it may increase your ability to bear challenging emotional states such as depression and prevent you from spiraling downward. Knowing your vulnerability, you may also want to enlist the support of a therapist early on, even in the absence of symptoms.

Dementia and Depression

You are not the only one who may fall prey to depression. The person with dementia is equally vulnerable. Although it is certainly possible to experience happy times while living with dementia, there are also many instances when depression is likely. For instance, depression is more often present with some particular forms of dementia, such as Lewy body dementias, Alzheimer's disease, and vascular dementia. Depression can also be a close companion of unprocessed grief and loss. To further complicate matters, some dementia symptoms overlap with dementia symptoms. For instance, executive dysfunction can lead to apathy and withdrawal from day-to-day activities, a common manifestation of depression. As the person closest to the one with dementia, you can be instrumental in noticing the possibility of depression, and in helping move the person out of his depressed state. Doing so will help save you both a lot of grief and keep the possibility of joy going between you. It is also one of the great gifts you can offer your loved one, noticing his mood and taking smart steps to help lift him out of his dark hole.

Assessing the Depression

The Geriatric Depression Scale is a questionnaire that is often used to assess depression in persons who are older and/or who have dementia. Answering the following questions will help you determine whether to be concerned about your loved one's mood.

1. Is he/she basically satisfied with his/her life?   **No**   Yes

2. Has he/she dropped many of his/her activities
    and interests?   No   **Yes**

3. Does he/she feel that his/her life is empty?   No   **Yes**

4. Does he/she often get bored?   No   **Yes**

5. Is he/she in good spirits most of the time?   **No**   Yes

6. Is he/she afraid that something bad is going to
    happen to his/her?   No   **Yes**

7. Does he/she feel happy most of the time?   **No**   Yes

8. Does he/she often feel helpless?   No   **Yes**

9. Does he/she prefer to stay at home, rather than
    going out and doing new things?   No   **Yes**

10. Does he/she feel he/she has more problems with
    memory than most?   No   **Yes**

11. Does he/she think it is wonderful to be alive now?   **No**   Yes

12. Does he/she feel pretty worthless the way he/she
    is now?   No   **Yes**

13. Does he/she feel full of energy?   **No**   Yes

14. Does he/she feel that his/her situation is hopeless?   No   **Yes**

15. Does he/she think that most people are better
    off than he/she is?   No   **Yes**

Each answer in bold above counts as one point. Add all bold answers for a total score. A score of more than five points is suggestive of depression and may warrant bringing your loved one to the doctor for further evaluation and possible treatment.

Thoughts and Happiness

The intuitive notion that thoughts greatly impact how we feel has been validated by findings at the University of California, Riverside. In their paper "Pursuing Happiness: The Architecture of Sustainable Change" (Lyubomirsky, Sheldon, and Schkade 2005), Sonja Lyubomirsky and her colleagues identify three types of determining factors of long-lasting happiness. Some are out of our control, but others are within the range of our influence.

Three Happiness Factors

1. Genetics: 50%

Our genetic propensity for happiness is set at birth and changes little over the course of our life. Indeed, half of our propensity to happiness is inherited, and there is little we can do to change that. That's the bad news for those of us with a "downer" personality.

2. Circumstances: 10%

Life circumstances contribute a surprisingly small part to our subjective feeling of happiness. Factors such as age, success, adversity, wealth, job security, income, health, and marital status turned out to have little impact on our well-being. The research found that people tend to adapt to whatever new circumstance, good or bad, befalls them. Positive events, such as getting married, or negative events, such as losing one's job, have the immediate positive or negative effects one might expect, but people soon adapt and revert to their original baselines. As a dementia caregiver, you probably can relate. With every new change, you may experience a temporary setback, a subjective decrease in your happiness, but eventually you have the potential to adjust to that "new normal." How you get there is where we turn our attention next.

3. Intentional Activity: 40%

Saving the good news for last: Forty percent of our happiness is under our control. And there are some specific steps we can take to cultivate it. "Circumstances" may happen to us, but we can choose to engage in intentional activities that influence and alter those circumstances. Mindfulness practice is one activity that can greatly improve your subjective sense of happiness. Through mindfulness, you can learn to recognize your thoughts and intentions and to discern which ones are increasing your happiness and which ones have the opposite effect. Then you can choose how you want to think and act in response to life events.

Overcoming Negative Tendencies

Even in the absence of depression, our human mind is still filled with a lot of negativity. Rick Hanson's (2009) concept of negativity bias is helpful to understand how our mind's negative tendencies are not just about us, but result from millions of years of evolutionary adaptation.

The Negativity Bias

When faced with negativity, we often blame ourselves for harboring such thoughts, thereby adding self-blame to our already unhappy state. Just as we do with the self-compassion break, or with the hindrances, we can help loosen the grip of self-negativity by seeing our negative thoughts as something larger than ourselves. We are negative because we are human, and our brain had to learn to protect us from life-threatening hazards.

> The alarm bell of your brain—the amygdala [...]—uses about two-thirds of its neurons to look for bad news: it's primed to go negative. Once it sounds the alarm, negative events and experiences get quickly stored in memory—in contrast to positive events and experiences, which usually need to be held in awareness for a dozen or more seconds to transfer from short-term memory buffers to long-term storage. In effect...the brain is like Velcro for negative experiences but Teflon for positive ones. (Hanson 2010)

Being a dementia care partner exposes us to many unpleasant stimuli and gives us many opportunities to react with negative thoughts and run away with a million stories. With mindful attention, each time this happens we can see our mind's inclination to "Velcro" to the negativity. Our emotional state gets easily flooded with the bad stuff and our good experiences get swept away. Because this tendency is greater than us, we need to take some concrete actions to help rewire our brain.

Rewiring Our Brain

We can rewire our brain to "Velcro" to positive experiences with a number of mindfulness practices. I invite you to try each one and see which one works best for you. We do this not just to "be positive," but because it is ultimately good for our mental and physical health.

FORMAL PRACTICE:
Taking in the Good

This practice was designed by Rick Hanson (2009) specifically to help us overcome our negativity bias. It is the practice of pausing long enough to appreciate good moments in our lives, so that our mind gets a chance to fully register those experiences. I have adapted it for the specific needs of dementia care. At first, you will need to do it sitting with your eyes closed.

- Think back on a pleasant experience you have had. It can be recent or many years ago. It can be small or significant.

- Revisit the whole experience: where you were, with whom, what happened.

- Notice body sensations, emotions, and thoughts that arise as you let yourself re-experience that moment.

- Instead of rushing through the memory, savor the experience. Let it fill your body and be as intense as possible. Focus on the rewarding aspects of the experience, whether it involves sound, sight, smell, touch, taste, or love.

- Savor the pleasantness and sustain it for a while, ten to thirty seconds. Don't let your attention wander somewhere else. If it does, bring it back.

After doing this practice, caregivers often marvel at the accessibility of such pleasantness. "I can call upon this good memory anytime!" This also helps you realize how malleable the brain is and how easy it is to produce positive thoughts and emotions.

Eventually, once you get the hang of it, you will be able to bring this practice into your daily life, including during shared moments with the person in your care. A great practice is to "take in the good" out loud with the other person. Sitting together, watching a sunset, you can share the goodness of your experience with your loved one and invite her to join in and share how that moment feels for her. If the person is nonverbal, you can still do this practice, relying more on a shared felt sense of pleasantness.

Half Empty and Half Full

When we are in the midst of the dementia care journey, our experience of loss can be so profound and repeated that our mind becomes habituated to being in a chronic state of grief. We fall into the habit of dwelling on wishes for what no longer is, while forgetting what can still be enjoyed. Bob, a student in one of my classes, drove the point home with this story:

It really hit me this week. I was standing next to Claire in the bathroom and noticed she no longer knew how to brush her teeth on her own. This was something new. Only the week before, she had still been able to manage on her own. I realized I had failed to appreciate that ability of hers while she still had it. I had been too focused on what she could not do to notice what she could still accomplish. In that moment I saw clearly that I could continue to proceed that way for the rest of our lives together. Or I could change, and decide to enjoy whatever we still have at every point. This was such an aha moment. I was able to do this because of what I learned in my mindfulness practice.

Can you be like Bob? Can you fully acknowledge your grief *and* also make room for appreciating what you still have going together with your loved one? Looking at both the glass half empty and the glass half full—with an emphasis on the latter.

Looking Around

During support groups, dementia caregivers often talk about what they gain from hearing others' stories. "Listening to other people in the group, I realize I have it pretty good. Things could be a lot worse." This is one of the benefits of getting out of yourself and taking the time to be out in the world: you can get in touch with the relativity of happiness. Whether it is other caregivers, the homeless at your street corner, the image of a child coping with cancer, or news about a distant war and displaced refugees, there is no shortage of misery for us to ponder. Doing so can help us put our own unhappiness in perspective. We realize suffering is all around, and part of the human condition. We cannot escape it, but we can certainly choose how we are with it. We may find inner happiness even in the face of extraordinary circumstances, including being a dementia caregiver. Looking around and opening our heart to the human suffering near and far is a great way to deal with self-pity.

Don't Expect, Be Happy

Connected with "looking around" is the idea of lowering one's expectations, an insight that naturally arose for me from spending time with dying and dementia patients. Contrary to what most people think, such work is not depressing. It is in fact quite the opposite. Being around those from whom all ends up being taken away gives one appreciation for everything, and I mean every thing.

Sitting next to Sue, a dying lung cancer patient, and seeing her painfully gasp for air with every breath, I learned to not take anything for granted, not even the ability to breathe effortlessly. Being around folks with dementia has made me grateful for the gift of my still-functioning mind. Seeing the effects of very old age on the body, I treasure each step I take, knowing that someday I too may need to settle for a wheelchair. I also savor my independence and the thrill of being my own free agent. I am filled with tremendous gratitude for whatever is given to me every moment.

Such appreciation can only come from having experienced the possibility of not having whatever it is we have in this moment. It is one of the gifts to be had from our experience caring for someone with dementia. Every mindful moment with the person can become an invitation to discover true inner happiness. We learn to treasure the simple things in life, and in the process we become less dependent on external factors to make us content. By lowering our expectations, we open the door for limitless happiness.

When Thoughts Get Sticky

The intentional cultivation of happiness is not enough. We still have to contend with habits deeply ingrained in our mind, sticky thoughts that won't quit, old stories, grudges, or unhelpful assumptions. Mindfulness helps us slow down enough to notice such traps, and recognize them for what they are. Mindfulness also gives us the tools to stay clear and find more freedom.

Recognizing the Problem

The first step toward letting go of persistent, troublesome thoughts involves recognizing them for what they are: mind habits to be dealt with just like any other habits. To let go of a bad habit, we first need to be convinced of the need to change the habit. Usually there is some kind of pain involved with the habit. We are overweight and our health is starting to suffer. The same applies to sticky thoughts. Ruminative, angry thoughts may consume us, and we find ourselves not feeling so good about ourselves as a result.

Second, we need to believe in the validity of the new habit and our ability to take it on. If I become convinced of the power of exercise and good nutrition, I will be more inclined to give it a try. With the mind, we need to find out for ourselves all the ways that our mind can work and that are helpful. When practicing "taking in the good," we realized how malleable our mind is. We need not be at the mercy of our automatic thoughts, and we can create well-being for ourselves, at will.

Helpful Solutions

Let's explore some different ways that we can help the mind get out of the rut it sometimes gets into with sticky thoughts.

FORMAL PRACTICE:
Going Neutral

This practice is a way of getting our mind to a neutral place. It can be done during either sitting or walking meditation. It goes like this:

- Let's say you have been thinking a lot about your neighbor and how lucky she is to have a healthy husband, unlike you. Acknowledge the thought and let it be.

- If you are sitting, put your attention on the breath. If walking, put your attention on each step.

- Whenever the thought comes in, no matter how often, acknowledge the thought and go back to either breath or step, as often as necessary. A thousand times if necessary.

- Notice your attitude toward the thought itself. Are you feeling annoyed? Do you wish it were not there? Are you judging yourself for being stuck with the thought? Are you experiencing unpleasantness and aversion toward the whole experience? Acknowledge that as well.

- Go back to observing the breath.

- Be patient with yourself and recognize the sticky thought as a mind habit. Habits take time to change, and habitual thoughts are no different.

INFORMAL PRACTICE:
Substituting Thoughts

Another way to abandon a sticky thought involves replacing the thought with another thought. Our mind can only hold one thought at a time, so while it is occupied with a different thought, the attachment to the persistent thought gets a chance to loosen.

- For instance, every time you start thinking about your lucky neighbor, consider holding instead thoughts of gratitude for what you do have.

- Every time the thought arises of *Kim is so lucky to have a healthy husband*, immediately go to *I am so lucky to have such a loving husband*, and contemplate a recent time when you felt love between you and your husband.

- Do not overthink this, and trust that the mind will rewire itself after a while.

INFORMAL PRACTICE:
Getting Out of Our Mind

Sometimes, the mind just needs a break from itself. The best way is to engage the other senses and practice sensory awareness as you learned it in chapter 5. Find something you can easily get into, such as gardening, swimming, playing an instrument, listening to your favorite music, or going dancing. The activity should be one that engages the body. Every time your mind wanders away to the obsessive thought, lightly acknowledge what happened and switch back to one of the other senses that is most called for in your chosen activity. Consider it another experiment with your mind.

When Someone Else Is the "Problem"

Our stickiest thoughts often involve another person. When we are faced with the extraordinary stress of caring for someone with dementia, our relationships may become challenged. A controlling husband may become more than we can bear when dementia gets added. Siblings may not be pulling their weight. And good friends may disappoint us with their lack of understanding or responsiveness. Our mind may latch onto a particular person and start building a whole story around him. The experience can be most unpleasant as we start carrying that particular person in our mind, wherever we go. To get some relief, we need to take action. Here are some proven ways to help disengage our mind:

Focus on the good qualities of the person.
If he has good intentions but falls short in his communication with you, focus on his intentions. If he has performed some good deeds, focus on that as well. Look for and magnify the good in him, no matter how small it may be.

Develop compassion for the other person.
Understand that his actions stem from his own personal suffering. Try to put yourself in his shoes and experience where he is coming from. While this is not easy, remember you are doing this for your own good.

Be practical, and accept your lack of control over the other person's actions.
You have two options. Either you continue to burden your mind with negativity or you decide to drop the thoughts. I have found it useful to reflect on all the previous occasions when I held on to grudges and angry thoughts, which were missed opportunities for peaceful moments. Now is the opportunity to change and drop the story, the same way you would drop a hot potato.

See the person as an opportunity to cultivate loving-kindness within yourself.
Seeing our mind react to the difficult person, and getting in touch with the resulting feelings in our heart and the pain associated with the whole experience, we may become more inclined to cultivate loving-kindness for that person. If we can come to a place of more love with that person, we will have paved the way for a more peaceful, loving mind.

Contemplations

Contemplation is a companion practice to mindfulness. Instead of paying attention to the present moment, we incline our mind to reflect on wise thoughts from various traditions or teachers. Contemplation can help bring agitating thoughts to rest. It can also take the place of mindfulness when we are too distressed to focus. Loving-kindness and self-compassion are forms of contemplation we have already explored. Let's add a few more.

Prayer

When your mind goes dark and there seems to be no way out, prayer can provide the opening you need. Depending on your faith, you may rely on familiar prayers from your own tradition. You may also contemplate the Serenity Prayer:

> (God), grant me the serenity
> to accept the things I cannot change,
> the courage to change the things I can,
> and the wisdom to know the difference.

The Serenity Prayer speaks perfectly to the predicament of the dementia care journey. No wonder it is such a favorite with caregivers in dementia support groups. The Serenity Prayer works equally well with persons with dementia, even late into the disease.

Four Remembrances

Sooner or later during your mindful journey through dementia care you will be faced with the wall of the reality of life's impermanence. You will have the choice to keep bumping your head against the inevitable, or to stop and contemplate the very nature of the wall itself. Whenever grief wells up inside, you may call upon these words, adapted especially for your predicament from a traditional Buddhist contemplation:

> I am of the nature to grow old.
> I cannot escape growing old.
> I am of the nature to become ill.
> I cannot escape becoming ill.
> I am of the nature to die.
> I cannot escape death.

Everyone and everything I love are of the nature to change.
There is no way to escape being separated from them.
There is no avoiding mistakes.
I am doing the best I can and I hold myself with compassion.

Dementia challenges us to accept each one of these truths. Strangely enough, while caring for my mother I used to find great comfort in telling myself those lines. It is as if the telling was paving the way for acceptance of what was to come, or what had already happened. May you too contemplate those words often. And may you too find comfort in them.

Clearing the mind is a lifelong pursuit, made even more necessary by our dementia journey. We have no choice but to try to keep our mind as peaceful as possible, so that we don't burden ourselves even more with our own mental fabrications. Clearing the mind is to be undertaken with great patience and compassion for ourselves. Now is not the time for added judgment, or for flagellating ourselves with harsh self-criticism. Instead, we can use mindfulness to notice our thoughts and steer our mind in the direction of presence, appreciation, and wisdom. That way, we put all the odds on our side and can minimize our chances of getting depressed or worsening our depression. Last, it is helpful to remember that we all suffer from negative mind tendencies. The same way we need to clean our house often to keep it pleasant, we also need to "clean" our mind so as to maintain ease and peace within.

Summary

Teachings

- Depression is an occupational hazard for dementia caregivers.

- It is important to evaluate your mental status regularly.

- Learn to recognize cognitive distortions common with depression.

- Look for depression warning signs.

- Take precautionary steps to prevent depression.

- Be on the lookout for depression in the person with dementia.

- We can rewire our brain for happiness with intentional thought practices.

Practices

- Formal practice: Taking in the good

- Explore: Half empty and half full

- Explore: Looking around

- Explore: Don't expect, be happy

- Formal practice: Going neutral

- Informal practice: Substituting thoughts

- Informal practice: Getting out of our mind

- Explore: Loosening thoughts about difficult persons

- Contemplation practice: Serenity Prayer or other prayers

- Contemplation practice: Four remembrances

CHAPTER 8

Learning to Communicate

Communicating in the presence of dementia represents a big challenge for both persons involved. For the person with dementia, brain changes have a pervasive effect on the ability to initiate and respond to conversations. It does not help that many of those challenges are not visible to the outside world. Unless we have a clear knowledge of the type of dementia involved and of the cognitive processes that go with it, we cannot decipher and understand the other person's attempts to communicate with us. And that knowledge is not enough by itself. In addition, we need to learn new ways of being with our loved one, moment to moment. Dementia requires that we make room for the person's differing reality, in addition to our normal, consensual reality. This is no small feat and cannot happen overnight. Only with practice, and many trials and errors, can we learn to relax into each moment and seamlessly move back and forth between both ways of being. In this chapter you will learn the foundations of mindful communication with the person with dementia, building upon practices and understanding you gained in previous chapters.

From the Person's Perspective

First, we need to understand how a person's ability to communicate becomes changed by dementia. Changes in language abilities, memory, executive functioning, visuospatial skills, and behaviors dramatically alter people with dementia's experience of themselves and of their environment. Comprehension and the ability to express oneself are also impacted. Furthermore, such changes are different with each type of dementia, and are likely to shift as the disease progresses. So many hurdles created by dementia in the brain are beyond your loved one's control. Through your conscious experiencing of what it might feel like, you get one step closer to truly communicating with him or her.

INQUIRY EXERCISE:
Changes in Cognitive Abilities

Let us take a look at the different cognitive domains and the changes within each domain that are common with dementia. In particular, we will focus on those changes that are most likely to impact the person's communication. As you go down the list, pause after each one and ask yourself the following questions:

- Does that apply to my loved one?

- If yes, pretend you are the one experiencing such alteration, and spend some time imagining what it might feel like.

- Reflect on how you may have responded in the past, and how you might proceed differently.

Language

- Stuttering or having difficulty pronouncing words

- Knowing the words but having difficulty getting them out, or not being able to get them out at all

- No longer knowing the meaning of words (for example, "What is 'fork'?")

- Having trouble keeping up with conversations or following directions

- Using many words to explain an object or an idea because you no longer know the specific word for it

Memory

- Repeating questions or statements because you don't remember
- Forgetting conversations, dates, or events

Executive function

- Not having it in you to initiate social interactions such as talking with family or friends, and relying instead on others to start conversations
- Staring into space for hours with no awareness of your surroundings
- Being able to hold a normal conversation one moment, then getting very confused the next moment

Motor

- Loss of expression in the face that can lead others to think that you don't care
- Slow, slurred, or barely audible speech

Visuospatial

- Difficulties moving the eyes that may lead you to stare in a way that feels uncomfortable for others
- Misperceiving objects, such as mistaking a wire for a snake and calling it that
- Not being able to recognize familiar faces

Behaviors

- Exacerbation of lifelong negative personality types, such as being overly critical
- Becoming irritable and mean
- Becoming disinhibited

- Losing empathy

- Talking continuously over other people

- Sexually offensive remarks or behaviors

- Hallucinations and talking about things that are not part of normal reality

- Having difficulty distinguishing dreams from reality

- Having sudden uncontrollable episodes of crying or laughing

- Repeating words or phrases

- Having abnormal beliefs that are not true

- Believing that a family member is an impostor

Mindful Communication Basics

In this section, we lay the foundation for sound communication with the person with dementia. First, we'll look at habitual ways of communicating that do not work so well. Then we'll explore a fundamentally new approach that can be applied to any situation, with any person, at any time. This way of looking at mindful communication borrows from Jon Kabat-Zinn's aikido communication technique as now taught in all mindfulness-based stress reduction programs. It is especially well suited for interactions with persons with dementia.

Three Ways of Communicating That Don't Work

At one point or another we have all engaged in one of the following ways of communicating with the person with dementia. While frustrating, such encounters can teach us a lot. These are common errors, so don't feel bad if you've relied on these to communicate with your loved one. The point is to recognize why they're unskillful and to learn new, more skillful ways to communicate.

1. Assertive

As the person with dementia comes to you with her different sense of reality and her particular need, you directly oppose her with your own reality or agenda. This looks like two people bumping into each other. Both end up getting hurt. This can be best explained with an example.

Ruth: "Can you help me find my husband?" [Her husband has been dead for several years and you know it.]

Reactive, assertive response: "I am sorry, but your husband is dead." [You respond to Ruth's request with what you know to be true according to conventional reality.]

Ruth's response: "Oh, no!... How come no one told me?" [She becomes very distraught at what feels to her like a devastating piece of news.]

Immediate assertion of your reality over the other person's experience results in stress for the person, leading to increased chances of challenging behavior.

2. Avoidant

Stuck in your reality, you don't like the person's request and you react by brushing her aside. It is as if the person were about to touch you, but you dodged out of the way at the last moment so that no actual connection was made. Common avoidance tactics include ignoring the person, changing the topic, or delaying the answer.

Reactive, avoidant response to Ruth: "Sure, but first how about some tea and cookies?"

This type of response only delays resolution. The person is likely to keep on repeating her question until she gets a response that meets her need. Repeated avoidance leads to frustration and distress.

3. Disempowered

You mean well and want to help the person. But you are stuck in your own reality and don't really know how to respond.

Disempowered response: "I understand—of course you want to find your husband. That must be hard not knowing where he is." [Stopping there and not being able to go beyond because you are wondering how to deal with the fact that her husband is dead.]

You are unable to help bring the person the resolution that she needs. That too can lead to distress.

In each case, we are hindered by our inability to effectively join the person and relate to her. We respond to her as we would to someone who does not have dementia. This results in an interaction that is frustrating for both parties involved. Fortunately, there is a better way.

INFORMAL PRACTICE:
Aikido Communication

Let us look now at how the aikido way can help us during our interactions with someone with dementia. The aikido way of communication draws from the Japanese martial art of that name. The aikido principle centers around aligning our energy with the person facing us. Applied to dementia, it translates into a series of four steps for the caregiver:

1. Set aside

Temporarily set aside your own agenda and reality, so that you can be fully present for the person. This includes temporarily letting go of any care task or any other thing you have in your mind and want to get done. Leaving your reality aside includes making room for the possibility of another reality, no matter how far-fetched it may seem. Whenever meeting a person with dementia, I empty my mind and ready myself for the unknown.

2. Enter

Enter the other person's reality:

- Take the time to clarify what the person is bringing, without assuming anything.

- Stay with the person's metaphors.

- Use all of your senses, including eyes and ears, to better grasp the situation.

- Bring your heart into this discovery, so as to understand the emotional need underneath.

- If you find yourself resisting the person's reality, simply acknowledge how you feel and let it be.

- Learn to play with "not knowing" and notice how you are with it.

With Ruth, entering might sound like this:

- "Sure, let me see how I can help you find him. Maybe first you can tell me where the two of you usually meet?"

Ruth told me about their time having coffee and a cookie "downstairs." I knew Ruth was used to having coffee with her visitors in the building lobby. I also knew her son was in town. Then it was easy to put the pieces together. Ruth was actually referring to her son.

3. Blend

Then, blend with the person's reality:

- Imagine the two of you holding hands and facing the same direction. This is the shift that needs to take place, from facing each other to turning around and aligning.

- Continue to stay in the metaphor to make room for the person's reality and also yours.

Continuing with Ruth:

- "Of course you miss him! You love him very much, and you wonder when you are going to see him next. Those times having coffee with him are so precious."

Notice how you are making room for both "husband" and "son" in your talk. Having joined her in her reality, you are able to relax and be fully with her.

4. Redirect

Gently but firmly, safely guide the person's next steps. Your willing stance has made it possible for the other person to trust you and join you.

Bringing final resolution for Ruth:

- "On the calendar, I see that you are due to go out with your son tomorrow. Would you like to call him to confirm?"

Next time you are with the person in your care, bring mindfulness to your interactions and practice setting aside, entering, blending, and redirecting. Go into it with a spirit of curiosity, and notice how the person responds. How did you feel during and after the interaction? What were some of the challenges, if any? This is about learning a completely new way of being with the other person, so you need to be very patient with yourself.

Mindful Responses to Common Communication Challenges

Repetitions

"Where am I?"

"We are at the doctor's office."

"Where am I?"

"We are at the doctor's office."

"Where am I?"

"We are at the doctor's office."

Memory Aids

None of us do well with repetitions. And yet with dementia we often have no choice but to listen to the same material over and over, many times. For some repetitions relating to the activities of daily living we can try to provide mental ramps for the person to better remember. The ability to read simple instructions is preserved until relatively late in dementia, and writing the answer to a common question can prove helpful. Some of the new technologies that provide real-time memory aids are also worth exploring.

Every Moment a New Moment

Most often, the solution is to be found within ourselves, starting with the mindfulness practice of welcoming each moment as a new moment, no matter how repetitive it may sound. As sensory awareness teacher Charlotte Selver (2007) put it:

> Every moment is a new moment, if we allow it. And every moment can be an old moment if we allow it. And you can choose how you can live with allowing new moments no matter how often you have to repeat yourself... So the question is whether to permit your nervous system a little bit more to be awake for the moment and moments you live. All the time, see possibilities of how you can be there this moment. Be there with this person, be there with this occasion, be there with this task.

Of course, getting to the point of seeing each repeated question as a new question is not easy. We quickly get annoyed and bored, the same way we might when we are practicing to be with each new breath. The person with dementia who keeps on repeating herself invites us to delve deeper into our mindfulness practice. Each new utterance of the same question can become the object of our awareness, the same way we have been practicing being with the breath or during mindful walking. The next time we encounter repetitions, we can say to ourselves: Aha, here is another opportunity to do my mindfulness practice. Let me see how I am with each repetition. Let me notice the automatic boredom response and the unpleasantness.

Compassion and Patience

Last, we get in touch with our heart, and we use compassion to step into the other person's experience. I find it helpful to remember my parking lot moments, when I have forgotten where I parked my car. That's what it's like for people with memory loss, only all the time. Their minds truly cannot remember from one moment to the next, and they need to rely on us for memory. If we can experience the memory loss with them, we are more likely to meet each new old question with more patience and love. As Olivia Ames Hoblitzelle (2008, 281) puts it:

> Repeated as many times as they were, listening to his repetitive fragments of conversation became a practice; I cultivated patience and tried to hear his words as if for the first time. Certainly I experienced plenty of boredom and frustration. Yet frequently I would feel a surge of love and compassion for him, realizing the enormity of what he was dealing with.

And when it gets to be too much, we can also give ourselves permission to take a break. Stepping out of the room, leaving to meet a friend, we can do whatever it takes to manage our sanity.

Alternate Realities

Hallucinations (seeing things that are not part of common reality), delusions (believing things that are not true), misperceptions (misinterpreting visual stimuli), and semantic difficulties can be equally challenging for dementia caregivers. We have no choice but to make room for such alternate realities. And we can rely on our mindfulness practice to be with what is—in this case, a reality brought to us by the other person, instead of our usual expectations of reality as we commonly know it.

Same Words, Different Meaning

Talking with persons with dementia, we may be misled by their use of words. The same word may not hold the same meaning for them as it does for us. Kate saying "My butt is drunk" is her way of communicating her need to be changed. We cannot take her words literally. Instead, we are invited to discover the inner poet within each of us and learn to play with metaphors. We temporarily let go of the strict rules of common language. Once we get the hang of it, this can actually become a rather joyful and playful experience.

Same Object, Different Sight

The former cancer surgeon looking at a series of black-and-white prints suddenly reminisces: "You have to be very careful when looking at those. It's very easy to make a mistake, and people can die," and he starts sobbing. With our deductive mind, we can see how the black-and-white prints may look like X-rays. And from the former surgeon's perspective, the prints *are* X-rays. Dementia loosens associations between words, memories, and visual perceptions. If we want to relate to the old surgeon, we need to relinquish our idea of shared visual reality.

A Better World

In many cases, the other person's altered reality has its own logic that makes perfect sense given the person's objective situation. I see this often in communal settings, where residents with dementia fashion the community according to their own needs and history. The former nurse thinks she is still working on the floor at the hospital. The former college professor thinks he is still in school getting ready to teach a class to the other residents. The elderly gentleman who had to leave his wife behind at home takes to his new neighbor and thinks she is his wife. I remember Betty, a socialite who had been used to a life of parties. Whenever she saw me, Betty used to tell me about yet another party she had to attend later in the day— "But I don't think I'm going to go. I'm not up to it today." Joining her in her confabulation helped her stay in a reality she could live in, as opposed to the unpleasantness of her situation in a modest board-and-care home.

Insects and Little Children

Dementia with Lewy bodies calls us to make room for the other person's reality, no matter how nonsensical it may seem. The main thing to remember is that that different reality is as real to the other person as our own consensual reality is to us. If we were in that person's shoes, dealing with the same physical changes in the brain, we too would live in that other world. The harmless little children who often populate the life of the person with Lewy body dementia are as much a part of that person's visual field as any of the "real" objects and people around. We, too, learn to make room for those little children as we join in, the same way we would when slipping into the imaginary world of Alice in Wonderland.

Behind each hallucination or delusion is an emotional subtext that we need to grasp in order to be able to effectively relate to the person. Hallucinations produce emotions, just as any "real-life" scenario would, and emotional needs may result in delusions, as in the case of Betty and her parties. With mindfulness, we learn to relax around whichever reality is part of this present moment. We suspend our judgment, and in the process make life easier for ourselves and the other person.

Beyond Words

Just as challenging is when the person has lost all ability to speak. I found this out firsthand with my mother after she suffered a massive stroke. On Monday, my mother was singing to me her favorite tune over the phone. On Tuesday, she had been robbed of her ability to speak. *Aphasia*, the medical term to describe what had happened to my mother as a result of her stroke, comes from the ancient Greek term for "speechlessness." It is associated with different types of neurological disorders, and comes in several forms. My mother was suffering from expressive (nonfluent) aphasia, meaning that she knew what she wanted to say but was unable to get the words out. Such a sudden loss is traumatic, and I had to rely on both my mindfulness practice and my field knowledge to be as supportive as I could for her.

Grieving for My "Talking" Mom

First, I had to deal with my own grief for the mother I knew who sang and spoke to me. Yet another loss down the path of Alzheimer's and very old age. We place such a high importance on others' words. In our mind, we equate relationships with the exchange of words, despite the now well-established fact that most of our communication is nonverbal. Our heart yearns for what we once had. With my mom, I had to give myself the space to contemplate and write about my loss. You may grieve in a different way, but the important thing is to not gloss over the loss of your loved one's "talking" self.

Voicing Her Loss

The loss of words is experienced by both sides. I needed to acknowledge directly to my mother what had happened and the likely emotions associated with the communication challenges that she was experiencing. When aphasia is complicated by memory loss, the person may forget what has happened to her, and this can feel extremely disorienting. One needs to be especially careful to not further isolate the person with a dismissive attitude. I made a point of telling my mother that she had had a stroke and was experiencing a temporary loss of speech. I wanted to keep her heart in a hopeful place, and there was indeed the possibility that she might respond to speech therapy. I also empathized with the extreme frustration she showed in her facial expressions whenever she was trying to talk, and I apologized for the times when I struggled to understand her. This is a step caregivers often forget in their communications with persons with aphasia. Even if such persons cannot speak or hang on to memories, this does not necessarily mean that they don't know what is happening in the present moment and cannot feel emotions. When we fail to relate to the inner process of such persons, we are actually further contributing to the alienation they are already feeling.

What's Left

In the absence of words, one is left to rely on two of the most profound forms of communication, touch and sight. Holding my mother's hand, I learned to look for her "squeeze" responses. Communication became very simple in its forced binary response. Yes or no. I like this, I don't like this... One gets down to the essentials of love and basic sensory awareness. Also, gazing into my mother's eyes, I shared some of the most tender and loving moments we ever had together. It was quite something to realize that it had taken that much for the two of us to get there. This is not uncommon. I have heard many tales of adult children who report a deepening of their bond with their parents following impoverishment of their loved one's language. One daughter told me she had never known the color of her father's eyes until the very end of his life, when dementia had rendered him completely mute. "My father's eyes are blue! I never knew the color of my father's eyes before." She shed tears from grieving over years of not really knowing her father until almost the end of his life.

The Gift of No Words

Being with my silenced mother, I found great comfort in recalling my own experiences of voluntary silence during long meditation retreats. Part of our discomfort with muteness in the other person comes from our ideas about what it must feel like to not be able to speak. We think it must be terrible, when in reality it may not be that at all. Once past the initial hurdle of giving up one's talking habit, one finds out that silence is actually a gift. Not speaking guards one from getting into trouble with wrong speech. Not speaking gives the mind an opportunity to rest more. Not speaking leaves more time for direct experience of the world around us. Not speaking is a relief. Not speaking also facilitates relating to others at a deeper level. I have always been surprised by the depth of connections that can be forged with other retreatants in the absence of any words exchanged for a week or more. Mindfulness practice prepares one to be at ease with the possibility of speechlessness both in oneself and in others. It trains us to give the other person the space to be in her speechlessness, without added pressure from our own discomfort.

Such profound ease around the person's muteness can have the paradoxical effect of creating the right conditions for the person to speak again. Stories abound of folks with dementia who start speaking intelligible words after months of muteness.

Is It Pleasant or Unpleasant?

I would like to share a little-known mindfulness practice that can make a big difference in how you live each moment. It requires paying attention to the quality of your experience. And it is remarkably simple! How we feel falls into three categories: pleasant, unpleasant, or neutral. Most of us don't stop long enough to notice, and yet this is precisely what we need to do if we are to maximize our inner happiness.

FORMAL PRACTICE:
Mindfulness of Feeling

1. Sitting down, eyes closed, get in touch with your breath and start paying attention to the quality of your experience. From moment to moment, ask the question: Is it pleasant or unpleasant? Do this for a few minutes.

2. Then, pay attention to how you react. Most likely you will find you want to hang on to the pleasant moments and to escape the unpleasant ones. This is how the human brain is wired. We are pleasure-seeking organisms.

3. Next, notice the accompanying physical sensations in your body, particularly places of tightness. Whenever we react to our experience, our body naturally responds by tensing the muscles. We each have a place that our body favors. For me, it is a knot in the stomach, but it could just as well be tightness in the throat or tension in the shoulders.

4. Without judgment, acknowledge any pain there may be. Pain is twofold, mental and physical. We stress our mind with our resisting thoughts, and we stress our body with our physical tensions. We can relax around this added discomfort and discover what a relief it is when we are just present for our experience, whether pleasant or unpleasant.

INFORMAL PRACTICE:
Mindfulness of Feeling in Relationship

We can take this practice into our daily life. During the course of my work with caregivers, I am often told that this is the one practice they have found the most helpful. Going through a tough moment with our loved one, we can relax in this simple acknowledgment of unpleasantness: *Unpleasant—this is unpleasant.* We also learn to see the transient nature of our emotional highs and lows: pleasant one moment, unpleasant the next one. That boredom, that annoyance, that pain shall pass, just like anything else.

We also understand the nature of things as they really are. Embedded in the pleasantness is the seed of ending and hence unpleasantness. Even the most pleasant things will turn to unpleasantness if indulged in for too long. To cling to the idea of constant pleasure is foolish. We need to lower our expectations and learn to welcome unpleasantness in our lives. That way, when it comes we are not surprised and we don't recoil with aversion.

We have little control over outer conditions, but we can definitely choose how to respond. Hearing Dad repeat himself for the hundredth time, we may notice the weariness in ourselves, and we can do a quick mental check: *This is unpleasant and I don't like it.* Making room for the whole truth of that experience, we are then free to move on.

Ending with this wise reminder I heard during a retreat I took with mindfulness teacher Ruth Denison (2010):

If you are not aware of the unpleasantness, it will snowball and leave the door open for more unpleasantness. If you are aware of the pleasantness, it will also snowball, but in the direction of more pleasantness.

Summary

Teachings

- Dementia has a profound impact on a person's ability to communicate.

- Communication is impacted differently by different dementias.

- In order to effectively communicate with the person with dementia, we need to first understand what communication must feel like from her perspective, based on her particular dementia, behaviors, and stage of the disease.

- We need to learn a completely new way of communicating in which we set aside our agenda and suspend our own reality.

- Mindfulness helps us meet various communication challenges, including repetitions, altered realities, and muteness.

Practices

- Inquiry exercise: Changes in cognitive abilities

- Informal practice: Aikido communication

- Formal practice: Mindfulness of feeling

- Informal practice: Mindfulness of feeling in relationship

CHAPTER 9

Responding to Distress and Challenging Situations

In this chapter we address one of the greatest challenges of dementia care: dealing with agitation and other forms of distress. Through mindfulness and careful tending of our heart, we can better prepare ourselves. Helpful heart practices include mindfulness of unhelpful emotional states, loving-kindness, and true compassion. We combine those practices with wise understanding of dementia-related distress and actions. We come to see most manifestations of distress as expressions of unmet needs. Special attention is given to frontotemporal dementia and Lewy body dementia, and the unique ways in which behaviors associated with both of those types of dementia need to be addressed. This mindful approach enables us to best attend to, and sometimes prevent, dementia-related challenges.

Responding, Not Reacting

When faced with irritants, the untrained mind is most likely to react, thereby missing the opportunity to find the space to choose the most skillful response. In ordinary life, such reactive ways can lead to unfortunate outcomes in work, relationships, and life in general. In the presence of dementia, matters are made worse by the other person's inability to mediate his words or actions. It is basically up to us to manage both the situation and our response to it. Getting angry at someone for yelling at us while he is hallucinating is not going to work. We need to find a way to manage our frustration and figure out the best way to respond. Most challenging is how to be in the midst of a situation where we don't have the luxury of contemplating our thoughts and emotions.

Mindfulness and Spaciousness

When I visit folks at the dementia care community, there is no knowing who will welcome me once the elevator door opens. Sometimes an angry resident is standing right there, and I have to respond fast and skillfully. Most helpful in that moment, when the other person is staring me in the eyes, is the calmness of my response and the internal pause I am able to find within myself. The agitated resident immediately relaxes, and we can both decide what to do next. Such calmness cannot be willed. It can only be the natural result of mindfulness practice or a calm temperament. Most of us need to practice this. I have found out the hard way, on those occasions when I showed up unprepared and too preoccupied to effectively meet those elevator moments. When dealing with dementia situations, mindfulness is a must, not an option.

INFORMAL PRACTICE:
In the Midst of a Situation

Make a point of sitting every morning and practicing. Next time you encounter a difficult situation, notice the "space" within. See what a difference it is making for you, and for the other person. Deconstructed, it might go like this:

- Take in the stimulus—in this case the words, actions, or the acute emotional state of the person.

- Find the space within where it can land.

- Take a breath.

- Relax any tension.

- Acknowledge unpleasantness, if any.

- Practice loving-kindness for yourself (and the other person).

- Keep going back to the breath.

- Respond to the situation in the best way possible, moment to moment.

More than anything, learn to appreciate the confidence that comes from knowing that you can rest safely in mindfulness. That awareness alone will reinforce your practice.

Understanding Distress

Challenging dementia situations have many causes. Understanding what is driving each one is essential to our ability to successfully address the problem. Some are common to all dementias and others are unique to specific subtypes.

Mindful Inquiry #1: The A-B-C Approach

Most expressions of distress come from an unmet need. It is up to us to explore with the other person the reason behind her distress. One helpful framework is the A-B-C approach developed by Marianne Smith and Kathleen Buckwalter (2006) specifically for dementia care. A-B-C stands for Antecedents, Behaviors, and Consequences. As care partners, we usually notice the behavior part first. Our first job is to pay attention to the unfolding of the behavior in detail. That will help us go back to exploring the possible causes of the behavior, the antecedents. The third step involves looking at the consequences, the ways we meet the person's behavior.

1. Behavior

When describing the behavior, think about the following:

- What is the person doing?

- For how long?

- How often?

- Where does the behavior happen?

- When does it happen?

- With whom?

2. Antecedents

Based on the previous answers, you can start looking in one of several directions for possible causes.

Physical Discomfort

When Peter approached me with great distress, saying, "I want to get the water out," I knew he was dealing with an urgent need. Only the words were failing him to adequately communicate it. I noticed him holding his crotch, and was able to make sense of what he was trying to say. Peter needed to go to the bathroom, and he needed someone to take him there, immediately.

Physical discomfort is the first place to look into when dealing with distress. The following checklist is a good starting point:

- Physical pain in different parts of the body

- Fever (warm to touch)

- Hunger

- Thirst

- Poor hearing

- Poor vision

- Uncomfortable posture

- Bathroom needs

- Fatigue

- Not enough exercise

- Uncomfortable clothing or footwear

- Skin tear or ulcer

- Difficulty breathing

Sensory awareness is the best way for us to elucidate possible sources of physical discomfort. Stopping to see, hear, touch, or taste—mobilizing whichever sense is most appropriate for the occasion—we put what we notice and our knowledge of the person together, and we come up with clues.

Environmental Stressors

In chapter 5 we touched on the importance of providing just the right kind and the right amount of sensory stimulation to the person with dementia. When a breakdown occurs in that delicate balance, the person is more likely to experience distress and act it out in the form of behaviors. Every time the noise level gets to be too much, we can be pretty sure Sarah is going to erupt into shouting her usual "Get me out of here! I wanna go home!" Besides excess noise, other environmental stressors to watch for include:

- Temperature (too hot or too cold)

- Light (too bright or not enough)

- Confusing patterns or mirrors

- Too many people and too much commotion

- Not enough touch, or too much, or unsolicited

- Television shows with alarming plots

- Unfamiliar setting

- Violation of personal space

- Triggering pictures, sounds, or stories

As with physical pain, sensory awareness is our best ally in our quest for possible environmental stressors.

Psychosocial Stressors

Most persons with dementia have a heightened emotional sensitivity and may react intensely to emotional distress, whether caused by external factors or driven by inner processes from the dementia. Psychosocial stressors include:

- Not feeling in control

- Not feeling useful

- Feeling excluded

- Depression

- Loved ones leaving

- Loneliness

- Picking up on others' negative emotional states

- People with negative associations

- Internal, from dementia processes such as hallucinations

- Disruption in routines

The more in touch we are with our own heart, the easier it will be for us to pick up on any one of those stressors as manifested by the person.

3. Consequences

Last, we look at how we responded to the situation. We do this without judgment, and in a spirit of compassion and learning. We understand that it is no easy task to relate to the dementia manifesting through the one in our care. We explore what worked and what didn't work. Through that inquiry we discover the causal relationship between our reaction and the outcome. The goal, of course, is to stop the need for the disruptive action. Often, when we are still searching our way through an interaction, our reaction turns into another trigger for further escalation of the situation. Examples of reactions that can act as further triggers include some of the unhelpful responses covered in the previous chapter on communication:

- Direct opposition to the person's words, usually with an aggressive undertone

- Avoidance or ignoring of the person

- Assuming the person has control over his actions, or trying to reason with him

More importantly, we learn to pay attention to the warning signs, the mini-distress responses that usually precede full-blown expressions of needs. This is when we have the time to figure out possible triggers and to do something about them. Of course, paying attention is what is crucial here, and mindfulness practice is our best protection against not noticing early enough. It is all really simple, once mindfulness is introduced as a matter of course.

Mindful Inquiry #2: Mindful Role-Plays

When all else fails and you can't figure out the cause of a recurring challenge, you can role-play the situation with a friend or another family member. Mindful role-plays are a wonderful way to empathize with the person with dementia. Over and over again caregivers have said to me, "I thought I knew what he was going through, but I didn't really know until I did the role-play. I came out with a much deeper appreciation of his needs." To get the most from a role-play, bring mindful awareness into the exercise. Here are some useful tips for embarking on a mindful role-play:

- Best is if you play the person with dementia in the situation, and someone else steps into the caregiver role.

- You may have a third person observing the two of you.

- This is not about doing a performance and trying to be an actor.

- You are simply trying to re-enact the person's words and actions in the context of the situation.

- The "caregiver" responds as you would normally.

- All along, the two of you should try to get in touch with the thoughts, emotions, images, and physical sensations that arise. The observer, if there is one, should do the same.

- After a few minutes, stop and process, taking turns listening to each other. I usually like the "person with dementia" to be the first to share, then the "caregiver," then the "observer."

- Go into this inquiry with an open mind and no expectations of outcome.

To give you a better idea, I would like to share one example of a role-play that led to some valuable insights for the caregiver.

Role-Play Vignette

Situation: Caregiver is getting frustrated with her husband, who stays up at night and insists on waiting for the van to take him to "the club." Her husband goes to an adult day program (the club) several times a week. All attempts to redirect him have not worked and only make him more agitated.

- Caregiver's insight during the role-play: "I got in touch with my husband's anxiety. I played my husband as he gets anxious even the night before, and he is waiting for the van to take him to the 'club.' It felt very real. While the other person was playing me and saying the same kind of things I usually tell my husband, I started feeling more and more anxious and frustrated. I did not feel she was taking me seriously, and she did not seem to be really listening."

- Other person playing her: "I felt really frustrated, and as if there were no solutions. I wanted 'him' to stop."

- Caregiver's insights after the role-play: "I realized I had not taken his anxiety *seriously* before. I just wanted him to stop asking. I got in touch with how much he likes going to the club. And I got to start thinking about what it is that he likes about the club. He likes to sing and listen to music. He also likes to call numbers during bingo. I realized he does not do any of these things at home. It's gotten pretty minimal, other than taking the garbage out and taking the dog for a walk. I now understand that what needs to happen is to give my husband the same kind of stimulation he gets at the day program. I can make sure he can listen to his favorite music. I can also explore more chores for him to do, so that he can feel more useful, particularly at night. One thing I need help with and I know he enjoys is sorting out the laundry."

Distress Questions and How to Answer Them

These questions are universal among persons with dementia. Word for word, these questions come to haunt us, with their insistence and emotionally charged quality. If we understand what triggered each one, we will be better equipped to respond next time.

"What Are You Doing?"

This is the person's way of telling us to back off. That question is usually triggered by a sense of losing control, of having something done to one without having been asked first. I once watched an old man being awakened without warning by a nursing aide, his sheets being pulled away and the aide reaching to loosen his belt so she could change him. The old man screamed, "What are you doing?" and started to kick and hit the aide. Anybody in his situation would have done the same. The best way to avoid such a response is to involve the person in decisions at each step. If we forget and our loved one reminds us with another "What are you doing?" we can always apologize, and thank him for reminding us.

"What Do I Do Next?"

You and I may appreciate idle moments here and there throughout our days. We may delight in not having to think about what's next. For the person with dementia whose executive functioning is compromised, not having a plan can be a source of extreme anxiety.

We need to hear the person when she asks, "What do I do next?" We do so by "lending" her our own executive function and by bringing structure into her daily routine. Best is a simple, factual answer about what is happening next, such as "It's lunchtime." Then, immediately follow with an empowering statement where she gets to exercise her decision making. "Shall we walk to the dining room?" Another, more structural way to help orient the person in time is through the use of new calendaring technologies specially designed for persons with cognitive loss.

"Can I Go Home?"

The person with dementia can feel estranged, even in his own home. In most cases, he does not mean going home literally. Rather, he is trying to get away from a stressful environment, and yearning for the comfort that is usually associated with home. Hence the emphasis should be on finding out what he is trying to get away from, and not so much on what he says he wants. There are several possible causes for such distress:

- The environment is too noisy, and he is not able to filter and process all the sounds coming at him.

- Routines are being disrupted, or he is in an unfamiliar place and literally not at home.

- He is with strangers.

- He is experiencing physical or emotional pain or discomfort.

I have found out that if you address the causes, the person will stop wanting to "go home." Home is in the heart!

"Who Stole My Purse?"

It can be incredibly painful having someone whom you are caring for falsely accuse you of stealing her stuff. Of course, she cannot help it. Memory loss is most often the culprit. She doesn't remember where she put her purse, then she looks for it and doesn't find it, and she jumps to the conclusion that someone, most likely you, must have stolen it. Most important is to not personalize the accusation. Once that's out of the way, you will be more likely to effectively address her concerns, remembering to practice aikido communication. You want to fully explore her mental landscape. This will help lower both her suspiciousness and her anxiety. You can then introduce the possibility that the item may have been misplaced, and that you can help in the search for it. Last, make sure to end on a reassuring note that the item will be found.

"How Can I Help?"

This question, and the agitation that may ensue if it is not adequately satisfied, can be hard to meet. Our idea of how to get things done, well and fast, does not go well with the often haphazard ways of the person with dementia. We may need to relax our standards, in terms of both output and speediness. Getting the house perfectly clean may need to take second place, behind creating a work partnership with our loved one. "Would you mind helping me vacuum the dining room?" A little effort toward making him feel helpful will go a long way toward the person feeling more content and less likely to have unmet needs.

"Where Is My Mother?"

The ninety-seven-year-old man who asks for his mother is not asking for his literal mother. Rather, he is looking to be nurtured in a very primal, immediate way. The descent into dementia can be terrifying, and asking for our mother is one of those instinctual responses that come to us under extreme stress. I usually validate the person's search for his mother, keeping in mind the actual meaning of his request. Singing familiar songs from his childhood may also provide some comfort. Even better is touch and gentle, firm holding, the same way you would hold a baby.

Less Common Situations and How to Approach Them

Next, let us look at some less common situations that can be associated with dementia. The first such set of challenges can be observed during delirium episodes.

Delirium

Delirium is characterized by a sudden change in mental status, usually in one of two ways. The person can either become extremely confused or agitated, or at the other extreme fall into deep apathy. The latter can be easily overlooked. Left untreated, delirium can lead to permanent, further deterioration in mental status. There are many possible causes of delirium, including medications, infections, and the stress from a foreign environment or extreme circumstances.

Hospitalizations

Hospitalizations are especially risky for people with dementia, and a very common trigger for delirium. Here are some suggestions for you to keep in mind if your loved one ends up in the hospital:

- Avoid or shorten hospitalization if at all possible.

- Try to spend as much time with the person as possible.

- Be as present as you can during each visit.

- Have a calendar with a schedule of your visits posted that aides can use to reassure the person.

- Make friends with the aides and nurses, compliment them on what they do well; they will be your most effective advocates.

- Coach the staff on the person's preferences and some key biographical information; type a list and have it posted next to the vital signs chart.

- Bring "home" to the room in form of family photos, flowers, favorite foods, a pillow or quilt, and familiar music.

- If at all possible, request a single room.

- Minimize distress from noise and commotion. Shut the door, and if it's a shared room, draw the dividing curtain.

- Ask for a room with plenty of light, if possible by a window.

- Give the person hope, and tell him he is going home soon.

- Keep reminding the person about where he is and why.

- Insist on involving the person in decisions made about him.

Infections

Infections are another common source of delirium, particularly urinary tract infection (UTI) and pneumonia. In the absence of any obvious physical symptoms, UTI should be one of the first things to check for. Care professionals in residential dementia care communities know this and are always on the alert for that possibility whenever a resident starts acting differently. Armed with that knowledge, you can do the same at home. Best is to call the advice nurse and suggest the possibility. Your loved one will provide a urine sample, and if it is positive, will be prescribed a course of antibiotics.

Travel

For those of us without dementia, travel can be an exciting opportunity to discover new cultures, new places, new languages, and new people. For the person with dementia, getting on an airplane and finding herself in a foreign place has the opposite effect. The dementia brain is not equipped to handle so many changes at once, and soon can go on overload. The results can be disastrous. I learned this firsthand during what was going to be my mother's last trip to visit me in the United States. Our newly recomposed family had just moved to a big brand-new home, it was Christmastime, and the house was filled with the laughter of our four teenagers with all their friends. My poor mother seemed fine at first, but within a few days she was hallucinating and in great distress. She became increasingly paranoid, to the point where I had no choice but to cut her stay short and send her back. Many years later, I witness other family members making the same mistake, over and over again. It is so easy to overestimate the dementia brain's abilities.

Not enough education is done on the high risk of delirium for dementia patients, which is unfortunate given how serious the possible consequences are, and also how easily it can be prevented if addressed early enough. Remember, any unusual and sudden change of mental status should raise your concern.

Frontotemporal Dementia

In frontotemporal dementia (FTD), many challenges are not due to environmental stressors, but rather come from cognitive changes inside the brain. The person with FTD who stops showing any warmth toward you is not doing so in response to something you said or did, but because her brain makes her. Equally difficult are compulsions and obsessions, such as constantly wanting food or hugs or needing to fill up glass after glass with water. Such behaviors are extremely hard on family members, who have no choice but to deal with them as best as they can. In this case family members are the ones experiencing distress, more so than the person with dementia. Mindfulness can become a saving grace for FTD caregivers. Here are some useful practices.

Wise Understanding

We understand that the behaviors of people with FTD are internally driven and not the result of unmet needs, as is often the case with other types of dementia. We also do not personalize such persons' behaviors, and we attribute their compulsions or lack of emotions to their illness. Such wise understanding can help us feel more compassionate, as well as to adjust our expectations of their behaviors.

Loving-Kindness

FTD is the ultimate test of our ability to love unconditionally, without any expectations of being loved in return. This is why loving-kindness for ourselves, and for the other person, is our best strategy when dealing with FTD behaviors. Getting there can be a long road, requiring lots of patience for ourselves and for the other person. Compassion practices, including the self-compassion break, can become ultimate refuges when all else fails.

Mindfulness

Mindfulness practice allows us to bring the calm presence we need when dealing with the constant behavioral challenges of FTD. Not practicing increases our chances of reacting, and thus of making matters worse. Mindfulness is also the practice that makes loving-kindness and compassion possible. Thanks to mindfulness of the heart, we get to clearly see the intricacies of our clinging tendencies, laid bare by the FTD care experience. Mindfulness shines the light into the darkest corners of our heart and opens the door for new possibilities within ourselves.

Skillful Limits and Redirection

When faced with impulsivity, disinhibition, compulsivity, and poor judgment, we are called to set firm limits, while preserving the person's autonomy and dignity as much as possible. We learn to tap into positive doors of engagement such as art, music, and exercise. Joining a community of other FTD caregivers can become invaluable. Thanks to technology, you can now find such support online.

Lewy Body Dementia

Similarly to frontotemporal dementia, Lewy body dementia (LBD) can be extremely challenging for family members. The challenges are very different, however, and tend to have more of a psychotic flavor.

Hallucinations

LBD hallucinations can strike at unpredictable times. The person may be fine one moment, and battling terrible demons the next one. When that happens, there is no reasoning with the person. It becomes most important to validate his reality while at the same time providing reassurance that no harm will be done to him. This may be challenging when he feels so threatened that he wants to lash out. While largely inner-driven, such hallucinations are more likely to be triggered or exacerbated by the following:

- Change in routines

- Too much noise and stimulation

- Lack of sleep

- Lack of exercise

- Not enough lighting, or confusing visual patterns

If the hallucinations are harmless (little children, aliens, insects), you may learn to make room for them in your shared life with the person. For rational types, this may prove challenging, but the alternative is not really an option. As we have seen in the previous chapter about communication, going against the other person's reality is bound to unnecessarily agitate the person. Mindfulness practice teaches us to be present for whatever is in each moment. If aliens are part of our loved one's experience right now, we learn to include them. This also applies to the persons with LBD themselves. Many times, persons in early stages of LBD who have a mindfulness practice have shared how their practice has helped them live with their hallucinations. They learn to live in a dual reality.

Similar to hallucinations, REM sleep disorder in persons with LBD makes it hard for them to distinguish dreams from reality. Violent dreams may get acted out during sleep. For the spouse, one practical way to cope may be to sleep in a separate bedroom. Consultation with a neurologist with expertise in Lewy body dementia should be considered.

Fluctuating Cognition

Lewy body dementia throws in an additional challenge for family members, in the form of constantly changing cognition. Caregivers will say, "My husband seems fine one minute, and all of a sudden he becomes completely confused. I never know what to expect." These constant unexpected changes can be extremely jarring to the caregiver's nervous system. Matters are made worse when the person has not been correctly diagnosed with Lewy body dementia, as is often the case. The ability to attribute cognitive changes to LBD can be a source of great relief to the caregiver, who can now be certain of the uncertainty in her loved one's behavior. Mindfulness helps us to avoid becoming attached to a certain way, starting by noticing what happens to us when we cling to an outcome. While it is only natural to favor those moments when our loved one is mentally together, with mindfulness we learn to recognize the hidden pain that comes with such attachment. We learn to more easily go with the constant back-and-forth between clarity and confusion.

Mindful Approach to Personal Care

Assisting with showering and toileting are two of the most challenging care tasks for dementia caregivers, mostly due to the situations that can serve as triggers.

Principles

Mindful care practices can make a huge difference, and will make the experience more enjoyable for both you and the person in your care.

1. Take the Time to Connect

- Sit with the person. As explored in previous chapters, taking the time to sit with someone signals to her that she matters and that you "see" her.

- Set aside your agenda and find out where the person is. Your agenda may be to get the person showered, but she may still be asleep and need time to wake up.

2. Meet the Top Two Emotional Needs

- Include the person at every step, no matter how small. You can start from the moment you ask permission to sit with your loved one. Showering involves many steps, and we want to transform the experience from something that is being done to the person to one that takes place with the person.

- Sometimes you need to be assumptive—for example, when the person's executive function is compromised. It may be time to assist the person to the shower. If that is the case, do state the task at hand, but immediately follow with a "yes" or "no" question so that the person still feels in control.

- Finally, make the person feel that he is assisting you as much as you are assisting him. Maximize his abilities, make him feel useful, and thank him for his help.

3. Relate to the Intimacy Challenge

- We each have our private zone. The needs for personal assistance in dementia require that we step within that private space. Even for couples with a history of physical intimacy, the interventions required often demand that we go one step further. Hence the challenge.

- During MBDC training, I have caregivers put disposable briefs on each other. Not until we actually experience what it's like can we grasp the full extent of the shame and humiliation of being subjected to such an invasive experience. The same goes with being given a shower or a bath.

- Armed with experiential awareness, we are more likely to bring true compassion into the way we assist the other person.

4. Be Aware of Cognitive Impairments

Challenges in different cognitive domains impact the person's ability to respond to personal care situations. By being aware of those different challenges, we will be better able to understand and assist our loved one.

• *Nancy's Example*

I would like to share an experience I had once with Nancy, a person with advanced dementia who suggested to me that she needed help with toileting. Once we were inside the bathroom, it was clear that Nancy felt overwhelmed and unable to decide on the next step. Visuospatial decisions are extremely difficult for a person like Nancy. She considered the sink, the toilet, and the garbage can, all receptacle possibilities in her mind. Nancy could no longer remember the specific function for each object. She had to be gently led to the toilet. "What do I do now?" As we have seen earlier in this chapter, such a question is indicative of impairment in the executive function, and requires an immediate answer. It was most important to break down the task into very small steps, and guide her through each one. In this case: pulling down her pants, pulling down her briefs, sitting on the toilet seat, doing her business, wiping herself, throwing the paper in the toilet, standing up, pulling briefs and pants up. Halfway in this process, Nancy got distracted and became obsessed with folding, unfolding, and refolding sheets of toilet paper. Such compulsive behaviors are indicative of damage in the frontal lobes of the brain. This required that I let go of my agenda. Nancy's urge had to be satisfied, and I became her assistant in neatly folding each sheet. She wondered where to place each "completed" sheet. We settled on the sink's edge closest to the toilet, and figured how to line up each sheet neatly. After a while, Nancy's agitation subsided and she became ready to wash her hands, another complex task. Stand in front of sink, turn on faucet, place hands under soap dispenser, soap hands, rinse under faucet, turn off faucet, dry hands with towel... Nancy appeared exhausted. Standing next to her, I found myself filled with an appreciation of the magnitude of the task, for both her and me.

Assisting a person with dementia requires that we let go of our agenda and step into another mode, one in which time and our need for efficiency stop. We do this with great compassion for ourselves, and for the other person also. And we make room for the inevitable impatience and frustration that will naturally rise within us.

A Complete Mindfulness Practice

So far you have learned a series of mindful sitting practices: mindful check-in; awareness of breath; the body scan; sensory awareness, including mindfulness of sounds; mindfulness of thoughts and emotions; mindfulness of feeling; and self-compassion break. The following puts them all together into one single thirty-minute practice.

FORMAL PRACTICE:
Sitting with Various Objects

Take your usual meditation seat and practice the following in sequence. Spend about five minutes on each object.

- Do a short body scan, starting with the feet and moving your way up.

- Then find the breath and practice awareness of breath.

- Switch to awareness of sounds.

- Notice your thoughts and emotions. Identify which hindrance may be present (anger, fear, or wanting what you can't have).

- Put your attention on the quality of your experience, either pleasant or unpleasant.

- Give yourself a self-compassion break.

- End with a few breaths.

  If and when you get lost, just go back to following the breath.

Summary

Teachings

- Mindfulness helps us respond, instead of reacting to behaviors.

- A mindfulness-based version of the A-B-C model can help to elucidate, prevent, and minimize challenging situations.

- Delirium, frontotemporal dementia, and Lewy body dementia present unique behavioral challenges and need to be understood and addressed differently.

Practices

- Informal practice: In the midst of a situation

- Explore: Mindful role-plays

- Explore: Mindful personal care

- Formal practice: Sitting with various objects

CHAPTER 10

Putting Yourself First

Each of the mindfulness practices you have learned so far in this book had the double aim of helping you best care for the other person while at the same time relieving some of your own stress. There does come a point, however, when you need to put the spotlight on just you. This is usually challenging for most caregivers. I have found that many wait too long to get the help they need. Guilt gets in the way, and before long, depression, frustration, burnout, and physical exhaustion set in. All the warning signs are there. You then have no choice but to finally put yourself first. Paradoxically, taking that step will make you a better care partner in the long run.

Body Basics

Self-care starts with the physical body. While true for all of us, this is especially true for anyone involved in the long-distance journey of dementia caregiving. By paying attention to the following body basics, you will put the odds on your side.

Exercise

I frequently hear caregivers complain that they don't have the time for exercise. To which I say, *not* exercising is *not* an option for you! Here are some suggestions for fitting exercise into your daily routine.

- Walk or bike instead of driving.

- Take stairs instead of elevators.

- Wear an exercise monitor to keep track of your steps.

- Whenever possible, include your loved one in your exercise routine.

- Inquire at your local gym, and look for the possibility of bringing your loved one with you.

- Start small, but be consistent.

- Find the type of exercise that is most enjoyable for you.

- Exercise with a friend, or join a class.

- Turn exercise into another mindfulness practice, just like mindful walking.

Another added benefit of exercise is its now well-proven role in brain health and possible prevention or delay of cognitive decline.

Diet

Also up there on the self-care pyramid is what we eat. Here is the list of priorities from the new preliminary dietary guidelines (*Scientific Report* 2015):

- Improving food and menu choices, modifying recipes (including mixed dishes and sandwiches), and watching portion sizes

- Including more vegetables (without added salt or fat), fruits (without added sugars), whole grains, seafood, nuts, legumes, low-fat or nonfat dairy or dairy alternatives (without added sugars)

- Reducing consumption of red and processed meat, refined grains, added sugars, sodium, and saturated fat; substituting saturated fats with polyunsaturated alternatives; and replacing solid animal fats with nontropical vegetable oils and nuts

To which I will add the practice of mindful eating that we explored earlier in the book. The less we engage in mindless eating, the more we will be able to eat just what we need to satisfy our caloric needs. We also need to be aware of the emotional aspect of eating. Too often we use food to compensate for our stress. I see that happen a lot with dementia caregivers. The more we can use mindfulness to process our emotions, the less likely we will be to resort to food.

Like exercise, a proper diet has also been shown to impact our brain health. Nutrition is important to reduce cardiovascular factors that can lead to vascular dementia and other types of dementia. We also know that diabetes and obesity are linked to greater risk of dementia.

Sleep

Caring for a loved one with dementia can have a severe impact on one's sleep. The reasons for such disruption are many:

- Depression and anxiety

- Stress and chronic hypervigilance

- Not enough exercise

- The other person keeping you up at night

We already explored how the body scan can be a helpful practice when you're lying awake at night, unable to sleep. Similarly, following the breath can be helpful. You may want to put your hand on your belly and focus on the rising and falling with each breath. If you are caring for a spouse with Lewy body dementia and find yourself kept up by his or her violent dreaming, you may need to part ways for the night and sleep in a different bed or bedroom.

Your Back

During the middle and later stages of dementia, when the person may rely on you for transfers and mobility, you will need to be especially careful of the damage you can do to your back from improper lifting. Take a class in body mechanics from an accredited instructor. It will be well worth your time. Layer that knowledge with mindful attention as you prepare to assist your loved one. Mindful assistance with transfers includes proper attention to your posture and taking the time to go through each step without rushing. It will also help to involve the other person and be true partners in lifting. Here are some pointers.

INFORMAL PRACTICE:
Mindful Transfer

- If the person is sitting or lying in bed, ask to sit with her first.
- Take the time to connect.
- Explain what you are going to do.
- Be aware of the person's state in that moment.
- Involve her in each step of the transfer.
- Talk through everything you are doing.
- Ask her to help you as much as she can.
- Express gratitude for her help.
- Check your base of support.
- Face the person you are lifting.
- Keep your back straight.
- Begin in a squatting position.
- Contract your stomach muscles.
- Keep the person close.
- Do not twist.
- Push or pull when possible.

Lastly, you need to recognize your limitations and seek assistance if necessary, including the possibility of home care or placement in an assisted living community.

Yoga and Mindful Movement

Yoga, tai chi, qigong, and other forms of mindful movement can be great adjuncts to your mindfulness practice. Importance is placed on the process, not the outcome. Practice to the best of your abilities while being careful not to hurt your body.

FORMAL PRACTICE:
Mindful Movement

Here is a simple yoga-inspired movement sequence I sometimes teach during my classes. All poses are done standing.

Mountain Pose

Stand as tall as a mountain, arms at your side, feet parallel. You may close your eyes if you want. Keep your shoulders down. Imagine an invisible thread pulling from the top of your head toward the ceiling, and another one pulling from the bottom of your feet into the earth. Find a place where you are perfectly centered, not too far back, not too forward. Play around with it. Meanwhile, continue breathing.

Neck Stretch

Let the weight of your head slowly and gently pull your head down toward the left shoulder. Keep the pose, and notice the stretch on the right side of the neck. Go back to center and repeat a few times. Then do the same on the other side. This is an excellent practice for those of us who spend lots of time on the computer or who are suffering from neck, shoulder, arm, or wrist pains.

Shoulder Lifts

Most of us tend to accumulate a lot of tension in our shoulders without realizing it. This exercise is a great releaser for the shoulders. Start by lifting the left shoulder as high as you can toward your left ear. Hold it and feel the sensations. Release, and notice the difference between the left and the right shoulders. Repeat once or twice.

Do the same on the other side. Then lift both shoulders at once and release. Notice the difference.

Horizontal Arm Stretch

Although deceptively simple, this exercise can feel very strenuous for those not used to exercising their shoulder and arm muscles. From just standing, slowly lift both arms on each side until horizontal, and hold for several minutes. Keep the shoulders down and stretch the arms as much as you can. Remember to breathe, and practice being with the physical sensations, including maybe some unpleasantness.

Standing Full-Body Stretch

Now raise your arms all the way up, as far as you can take them without lifting your shoulders. Again, keep that pose for as long as you can, and remember to breathe. Stand as tall as you can.

Side-Bending Stretch

From full-body stretch, bend from the waist toward the left side. Only go as far as your body safely allows. Keep facing the front of the room. Keep your shoulders down. Go back to full-body stretch. Then repeat on the same side. Then do the other side. While you are doing this pose, consciously breathe, and notice the movement of breath within your body.

Standing Twist

Raise both arms to a horizontal position, then, keeping the arms up, rotate from the waist toward the back of the room. You can use your gaze to direct you, looking as far back as you can. All along, keep your shoulders down. Remember to breathe, and notice the effect of each breath on the internal organs while you hold the pose. Only go as far as your body allows. Repeat once or twice, then do the other side. Another variation of the same pose involves rotating the whole body from the hips up. Notice how, this time, the sensations become even more pronounced.

Chair Pose

From the mountain pose, pretend you are sitting down on a chair, and go down as low as you can. Then raise your arms forward as far up as you can, while looking ahead, keeping your shoulders down. Hold the pose. Repeat a few times. The chair pose is an excellent preparation for times when you need to assist with lifting or transferring the person in your care.

Mountain Pose

End with the mountain pose. Focus on the in-and-out movements of the breath.

If so moved, you may transition to a formal sitting mindfulness practice, awareness of the breath, or any other favorite. Mindful movement is a great preparation for mindfulness meditation practice.

Getting Help

It does take a village to care for a loved one with dementia. The more you can lean on others, the more you will disperse the stress. Now comes the hard part of asking for help. The biggest hurdle seems to be a mental one. A common misconception with caregivers lies in the belief that in order to be full-fledged caregivers, they need to do it all. The admission of needing help is only made reluctantly and after much inner turmoil. It is a process that often cannot be rushed. I just want to tell you this: asking for help is a sign of strength, not weakness.

Turning to Experts

Experts in care are all around you. Here are a few places to start.

Free Care Management Resources

Only one phone call away are experts you can turn to who won't cost you a dime. Your local Area Agency on Aging (AAA), the Alzheimer's Association, and other advocacy organizations specific to the type of dementia you are dealing with are great resources. The AAA can point you in the right direction for legal and financial matters such as long-range planning and estate planning. They can also help you get help with driving evaluations, home modifications, and other safety measures. Social workers at senior centers and adult day programs are other often untapped resources.

Geriatric Care Managers

Geriatric care managers can save you a lot of grief, and in my opinion are well worth the expense. A geriatric care manager can help put in place a personalized care plan for you and your loved one. This person can also provide ongoing care management if you can afford it, relieving you of many headaches along the journey. The National Association of Professional Geriatric Care Managers is my go-to place.

Support Groups

Last, support groups are not just there to help you emotionally. You will find other group members and also group facilitators filled with helpful knowledge about every aspect of dementia care. Most important is to find a group that is relevant to your situation in terms of dementia type and stage.

Getting Respite

If and when you are ready for help, you may consider the following options.

Friends and Family

You will need to know how to ask for help. Be specific as to the kind of help you need, and leave the door open for a refusal. Some websites are making it easier. You can invite your friends and family to join, and then post any request for help as problems arise. Here, you are being asked to practice receiving, as opposed to just giving. You'll be surprised how easy it becomes over time. Your asking for help from many is good not just for you, but for those on the giving end. It is in fact building a community of care. Such a community will sustain you over the years during your dementia journey. Even if you do not have a large family to draw on, you can start with neighbors, friends, volunteers, and other caregivers you meet in support groups.

Home Assistance

When more care is required, home aides may be your best option. But you should be aware that if there are other people in your household, bringing a stranger into your home may cause them some trepidation and discomfort. The person with dementia may also resent having someone new brought in. Know that home agencies are there to help you. Your most important role is in picking a reputable agency and vetting the personnel they send to help. Start with a few hours one day a week and see how it goes.

Adult Day Programs

Adult day care and adult day health programs are one of the most underutilized resources as far as dementia care is concerned. And yet those types of services can be life-changers for both family caregivers and the people in their care. Adult day services provide socialization, structured engagement, care oversight from specialized staff, and ongoing support for families. Family members also get much needed respite. Lastly, such services have the advantage of being a relatively affordable option, and they can often delay the move to assisted living. I am a huge fan of adult day programs.

Residential Care

When you can no longer keep your loved one at home, residential care then becomes the best option for you and the person. Take your time to find the right community. When dementia is present, I usually recommend that you pick a community specifically designed to cater to the needs of persons with dementia. You can look at assisted living communities or board-and-care homes. The latter are usually cheaper than assisted living and have the advantage of offering more of a home setting. However, they are often lacking in terms of providing meaningful engagement. One possible option is to supplement board-and-care living with adult day services.

Temporary Respite

Sometimes you may just need a break. Going away for one or several weeks, alone or with friends, can do wonders for your mental health. One little-known fact is that many residential communities offer temporary respite. This can actually be a good way for you and your loved one to try things out before committing to a more permanent move.

Seeing a Shrink

The dementia care journey ranks way up there in terms of the stressors and challenges involved. Yet very few caregivers end up taking advantage of the counseling opportunities that are available to them. That is unfortunate, and I would like to encourage you to consider this if you have not yet done so. Don't wait until depression sets in. A therapist can help you with many issues along the way, including mild depression, grief, couple and family issues, and ongoing stress.

When Love Is Not There

Not all adult children or spouses feel love toward their relative with dementia. A whole history of hurts may be present that needs to be contended with, and dementia only serves to magnify the truth of a damaged relationship. What to do then? So much judgment is attached to how a child (particularly a daughter) or a spouse (particularly a wife) is supposed to behave. Spouses who have been cheated on or who have suffered from an abusive relationship are now being asked to put their life on hold to care for their partner. For many, that is too much to bear, and providing care from a loving place is simply not possible. Mindfulness practice can become a great inner resource for such families.

Letting Go of Judgment

Mindfulness helps us make room for all possibilities, including the absence of love or the presence of difficult emotions such as anger, resentment, or even hatred. And we can make room without judgment. The more accepting we become of the hardness or unease in our heart, the more we will be able to feel compassion for ourselves, and eventually for the person we are responsible for. Then the work becomes to accept one's limits and to put in place other ways to provide the person with the care and love he or she needs.

A Change of Heart

There is also always the possibility of a change of heart. All the practices learned in chapter 6 can be used to investigate the heart, and to explore ways that may enable us to soften and forgive past misdeeds. We do this for the other person, but even more for ourselves. A tight heart is not good for our health and it is worth trying to ease it as much as possible. That much we can do.

Mindfulness

Of course, the kinds of daily, formal mindfulness practices that you have learned in this book are best for your mental and physical health. Thirty minutes every day is ideal. I would like to add the following two suggestions to your mindfulness toolbox.

FORMAL PRACTICE:
Bookends

Similar to STOP, this is a short yet powerful practice. It goes like this.

When you wake up:

- Before you get up, keep your eyes closed.

- Follow your breath for a few moments.

- Notice where you are in terms of feelings, emotions, thoughts.

- *Then* get up.

- This is your chance to start the day with a mindful attitude.

When you go to sleep:

- While lying in bed, practice loving-kindness for yourself.

- And then practice loving-kindness for the people you encountered during your day, including those with whom you experienced difficulties.

- If you prefer, you can practice giving yourself a self-compassion break instead.

- This will allow you to bring a calming closure to the end of your day.

Daylong Retreat

Eventually, you may want to do a daylong retreat. Such retreats are now commonly conducted in many places, including traditional meditation centers. Although the prospect of practicing for a whole day may seem daunting for mindfulness newbies, I yet have to come across any participant who did not benefit in the end.

What to Expect

- All practices will be done in silence.

- You will get an opportunity to share with the group at the beginning and the end.

- Most practices will be guided.

- A teacher will be available throughout the day to privately answer your practice questions.

MBDC Daylong Example

- Welcome, 15 minutes

- Body scan, 30 minutes

- Sitting, 30 minutes

- Walking, 30 minutes

- Sitting, 30 minutes

- Mindful lunch, 60 minutes

- Walking, 30 minutes

- Loving-kindness, 30 minutes

- Walking, 30 minutes

- Sitting, 30 minutes

- Group sharing, 30 minutes

- Mindful closure, 15 minutes

How to Prepare

- Get plenty of sleep the night before.

- Make a point of arriving on time.

- Dress in comfortable clothes.

- Bring your favorite blanket and pillow if you want.

- Bring lunch, snacks, and a water bottle.

- Most importantly, come with an open mind.

- Think of the day as a succession of individual moments.

After the Retreat

- Take time to process and take in what you have learned from your day of retreat.

- Minimize social contact and activities the evening after the retreat.

- Do not be surprised if you feel tired for a few days afterward.

- Use the momentum gained during the retreat to infuse your practice with renewed energy.

With retreats we get to value the gift of sustained silence and quiet inner listening. The longer the retreat, the longer the benefits will last. I was moved to write the following poem at the end of a two-week silent retreat.

Silence gives one the space
to notice one's own thoughts.
Silence puts one in touch
with the reality of the heart,
whatever it might be.
Silence makes it easier
to watch one's actions.
Silence protects one
from oneself.
Silence of the human kind
allows other living things
to have a voice again
—the birds, the air, the insects…
even silence itself.

I wish you to discover the gift of mindful silence also…

Summary

Teachings

- Self-care is not just for you, but also to help you sustain your journey as a care partner.

- Self-care starts with the body: exercise, diet, sleep, watching your back, yoga and other mindful movements.

- Many self-care body routines are also good for your brain.

- Getting help is a sign of strength, not weakness.

- Resources are there for you to access if you want.

- When love is not there, mindfulness can be your greatest ally.

- Going on a full-day retreat will help deepen your mindfulness practice.

Practices

- Informal practice: Mindful transfer

- Formal practice: Mindful movement

- Formal practice: Bookends

CHAPTER 11

Reaping All the Fruit

You have been practicing mindfulness every day, by yourself and also during your care interactions. By now the fruit of your mindfulness practice may have started to reveal itself more fully. You may notice a difference in how you are with yourself, the way you are with the person with dementia, and that person's response to you. This attitudinal shift leads you to view dementia not just as a challenge and a long good-bye, but also as an opportunity for growth and a deepening of your practice. You can also use mindfulness practice to help you relax rigid, maladaptive ideas of yourself and move to more fluid roles based on what is required by your loved one in the moment. In this last chapter, you will also get a chance to review what you have learned in the book and to formulate a plan for moving forward.

Two Last Things

If You Are Far Away

This book would not be complete without addressing the special situation of long-distance caregivers. Being a long-distance caregiver is hard, especially when a loved one's mind can no longer dwell on the memory of prior times together or the anticipation of a future visit. One can easily feel helpless and overcome with grief and guilt and frustration. Fortunately, thanks to modern communication devices, there are simple ways through which you can stay connected. I want to tell you a story about my mother.

Given that I lived five thousand miles away from her, my contact with her was mostly in the form of short daily phone calls. At first I wondered, *What's the point? A few minutes can't possibly make a difference.* And then one day I had to go on a long vacation without easy access to the phone. I did not call my mother for three weeks. When I returned, I learned from my brother that my mother had been out of sorts during my absence. After a few days of my resuming my calls, her agitation subsided and she was back to her normal self. My daily calls did make a difference in my mother's heart.

If you are a long-distance caregiver, take advantage of the phone or other communication devices to give your loved one the gift of your mindful presence. Here are some tips.

Be Consistent

People with dementia have a keen internal clock, and routine is extremely important. That routine can include your daily call.

- Better to have daily contact, even if very short and on the phone, than to spend a whole day with your loved one and then not have any interaction for three months.

- I have found that establishing a connection usually carries the person throughout the day. By the next day, however, the effect has dissipated and it is time to recharge the person's heart with some more reassurance and love.

- Call at the same time every day. I timed my calls at 8:30 every morning, just in time to catch my mother before dinner in France, where she lived.

Be Fully Present When You Call

The words almost do not matter, but your authentic presence does.

- Before making the call, free your mind from all your "stuff."

- Fill up your heart with loving-kindness, readying yourself to be with your loved one. I visualized my mother's face and I smiled before I picked up the phone.

- Sit down while you talk, and be wholeheartedly engaged in your conversation and nothing else.

- Treat each call as a brand-new call, no matter how repetitive it may seem from one day to the next.

Pack Your Talk with Emotional Goodies

Touch upon your loved one's emotional needs all at once.

- Start by giving the person a chance to make a decision about your conversation. "Is this a good time to talk?"

- Stick to safe topics that don't test memory and that preserve self-esteem. "What is the weather like where you are?" "How is your health?" "How are you feeling?" Keep the conversation simple.

- Volunteer material and bring in good news. I used to talk to my mother about my daughter and how well she was doing in college.

- End with an affirmation of your love and a reassurance that you will reconnect the next day. "I love you lots, Mom." When she reciprocates, tell her how good it makes you feel to hear those words from her.

- Also emphasize how much you needed to talk with her and what it brought you. That way you make her feel that she still has a role to play as your mom.

Don't Get Hung Up on Reality

With my mother, I learned to let my imagination run wild, and say anything that would leave a positive impression in her heart.

- My mother probably did not remember the exact content of my talks with her, but she remembered the emotion. That I loved her, and cared for her, and was a constant in her life. That there were still things for her to look forward to. That she could still treat me to lunch, even though it had been years.

- "When are you coming?" she would ask. At first, I used to be accurate in my response, but I soon found that three months felt like an eternity to her. After a bit of playing around with the truth, she let me know that one week was just fine. "I am coming next week." "How long will you be staying?" she would always ask. And each time, I answered, "One week." That brought her so much happiness. Such a small thing, but it meant so much to her! I was able to do that, every day.

In the End

When the time comes for the final parting with your loved one, you may apply the same mindful presence that sustained you throughout the dementia. And also:

Stay Calm

One possible response to a loved one's dying is to become anxious and engage in various activities. This can be upsetting to the dying person and add to his distress. Better instead is to calm yourself down, and bring the gift of your quiet presence. Remember, this is not about doing for the person but rather being with him. Sit quietly and tune in to your breath. Read him a favorite scripture or poem. Hold his hand. Gently massage his feet.

Do Not Argue

In cases when the person becomes restless and wants to get out of bed, do not argue. Rather, reassure him with a calm voice and decrease any unnecessary stimulation that could increase the restlessness. Holding his hand and gently stroking it may also help lessen the agitation.

Act as If the Person Can Still Hear

Even if the person appears unresponsive or speaks in a way that does not seem to make sense, refrain from talking in the third person. Do not share information that could be upsetting or disrespectful. The sense of hearing is the last one to go, and stories abound of dying ones who surprise their families with unexpected bouts of clarity.

Follow the Person's Lead

Some people want to be touched, while others don't. A frown, a pulling away of the hand are signs that the person is withdrawing and prefers that you not touch her. Same with playing music and with other sounds, smells, visitors, and so on. Sometimes the person can tell us if that is something he wants. If not, we need to pay attention to nonverbal ways of communicating.

Keep Family Quarrels Out

More than once I have seen family members fight over inheritance, or over the ways that their loved one's death and dying should be handled, right by the bedside. Such quarrels create unnecessary distress for the dying person. If possible, be an advocate for the person and ask your family to have the discussion somewhere else.

Ease the Physical Pain

Respect the hospice team's decision regarding which and how much pain medications to give. Your loved one's comfort is at stake. If it looks like your loved one is in pain still, signal this to the nurse in charge, and explore ways to maybe increase the medication.

Hold Off on Food and Drinks

Although we are used to equating caring with offering food and drinks, in this case we need to shift our view to make room for the reality of the dying one. As the body shuts down, the requirements for food and drinks progressively stop, and it becomes important to not get in the way. Do not force water intake. You may try to drip a few drops of water from a spoon, or hydrate his tongue with a small sponge soaked with water. You can also moisten his lips with some lip balm.

Do Not Be Surprised by the Look and Sound of Death

Be prepared for changes in the way the person breathes, interacts, feels, and looks. The death rattle can be scary to hear if you have never witnessed it before. So is the sight of glassy, half-open, tearing eyes, and the touch of a stiff body, cold as stone. You need to know that these things are not painful but rather normal physical manifestations of near death.

Spend Time Contemplating the Inevitability of Death

The Buddha advised us to say this to ourselves: *All that is dear to me, and everyone I love are of the nature to change. There is no way to escape being separated from them.*

A New Attitude

Practicing mindfulness, one realizes that the key to finding joy, even in the midst of challenging circumstances such as caring for a loved one with dementia, lies not in external changes over which we have no control, but rather in our growing ability to shift our attitude and our way of being in the world. Such a change can be hard to grasp and articulate, but you will know when it happens.

Relaxing the Self

The way we think about ourselves, and about our roles in relationship to others, has a profound influence on how we approach and experience the person with dementia. Our usual ways of identifying with predetermined roles and expectations can get us in trouble if we are not careful. With practice we can learn to navigate between two realms: the constructed self and the essential self.

The Constructed Self

The "constructed self" refers to fixed ideas we have constructed over time about our sense of self, which include:

- The way we present ourselves to the world, including our name, our professional identity, our traditional family roles, and our personal history

- Our expectations of how others should behave and respond to us and others, their names, their personalities, and their assumed relationships to us

- Memories of the past and expectations about the future

Example: *I am my mother's daughter, and that will never change.*

The constructed self is what allows us to function in the world. The constructed self also shows up during our formal mindfulness practice, in the form of automatic thoughts about "me" that have nothing to do with the present moment. These thoughts are usually about sticky identities of ourselves that keep on intruding even when they're not relevant to the present-moment experience. For instance, as I am sitting watching my breath, all of a sudden a thought arises about "me" that has nothing to do with the present moment. I may start thinking about needing to prepare for a work meeting. This is an example of the constructed professional self manifesting. Other ways to talk about the constructed self include "functional self," "storied self," and "conceptualized self." You may have your own word for it.

As Olivia Ames Hoblitzelle (2008, 55) puts it:

We freeze everyone into a complex of fixed concepts about "who they are," or at least who we think they are. We assume familiar, predictable patterns of behavior. We spin a world of concepts, expectations, and assumptions, and then live relating to the world of our own creation more than to the reality of the person as he or she is in this moment. When a piece of carefully constructed reality falls away, we're caught unawares. We're left momentarily empty. "Where is he?" "What's going on here?"

The Essential Self

The essential self is not a fixed thing, but rather a way of being from moment to moment. We dwell in the essential self whenever we ask ourselves questions like these:

- What is needed in this moment?

- What does the other person need from me?

- How does she view me, and what is the most compassionate response?

Example: *Right now, in this moment, I am being her sister because that is how she now thinks of me. I relinquish the idea of her as mother and me as daughter.* We can draw inspiration from Christine Bryden, herself a person with dementia (2005, 152):

> *Living in the present is where our true self is... I now know that in this journey towards my true self, with dementia stripping away the layers of cognition and emotion, I am becoming who I really am... All we can do is intensely experience the now of each moment with you. Treasure these moments and you will be able to share true acceptance of self.*

Back and Forth

The essential self is what allows us to relate to the person with dementia, particularly in the most advanced stages when the person's constructed self has eroded the most. During meditation, we dwell in the essential self whenever our attention is right there with the breath, and the body sitting, and the hearing of sounds, and nothing else. We are experiencing the moment instead of thinking it. We can then bring this way of being into our interactions with the person with dementia. Conversely, we learn to appreciate dementia interactions as opportunities to further discover what it's like to operate from the essential self.

And of course, we also need to bring in the practical reality of our constructed self, as when we provide gentle redirection after entering into and blending with the other person's reality. This is not a case of either/or, but rather of fluidly moving between both experiences of one's self based on the requirements of the situation. What is your story as it pertains to your sense of self? Think about roles you identify with most often, including during your interactions with your loved one with dementia. And then do the following practice.

FORMAL PRACTICE:
Sticky Selves

The next time you sit with the intention of following your breath, notice each time when your mind wanders. Make a mental note of the object of each wandering. Then go back to the breath. At the end of your practice, recapitulate all your wanderings. How many, if any, involved an aspect of yourself, a role, an identity? Were you being a wife, a husband, a daughter, a mother, a teacher, a gambler, a helper? The more you do this practice, the more you will be able to see the stickiness of such self-identities, and how such thoughts get in the way of being in the moment. Self-related thoughts are also usually the cause of much stress. The more we are able to temporarily abandon such thoughts, the more we will find peace and ease during our practice. Starting to observe first while sitting makes it easier to see the mind at work. Eventually we can transfer this practice into our activities of daily living. You can even make it a game, and name all the different personas in your world. Being with your loved one with dementia will present you with innumerable opportunities.

The Other Side of Grief

The other major shift that takes place with mindfulness lies in our ability to experience grief differently. At first we may have felt consumed by ongoing grief in ways that we may not have even been aware of, as we saw in chapter 3. Over time, however, we eventually learn to make room for and recognize all the emotions that are part of our grief process. And we get to see grief as a source of much wisdom.

What Grief Can Teach Us

Grief, as I have come to understand it, is also an extraordinary opportunity to experience and see close up the suffering caused by clinging in its most extreme manifestation. Here I would like to share with you my mother's parting gift, in the form of notes from an encounter I had with her shortly before she died.

Yesterday, when I arrived, I found her sitting at her usual table in the back of the dining room. Remembering our intense connection from two weeks ago, I expected at least an acknowledgment, a gaze of recognition, a smile. I was met instead with a blank stare. I sat by her side and waited. "Bonjour, Maman. C'est Margot, ta fille." She looked up, gave me a look, and closed her eyes again. Aides had laid out dinner in front of her, and I was to help her. It took forty-five minutes for her to get one serving of Ensure down. I followed the aides as they wheeled her back to her room, and I kept her company as she lay resting in bed. Giving her kisses, stroking her forehead, reaching out for her shriveled hand did not produce the usual joy in her. Rather, it became clear that she wanted to be left alone. She is withdrawing from the world, I thought, and she is letting me know.

My mother mostly wants to sleep, and sometimes drink a little, that's all. No more music, no more engagement, no more closeness, no more food. This is in direct contrast to the mother I knew, who loved singing so much, and eating well, and being hugged and cajoled. That version of her no longer exists, other than in my memories, which are thoughts about the past with no relevance to the present conditions. Turning inside, I get in touch with the pulling away and the hanging on from lingering grief. What we call "love" is first and foremost attachment. The more we feel love, the tighter the bond, and the more difficult it is to let go of the object of our love. True love is purified from all attachment, and demands that we not burden the loved one with the imposition of our clinging. It also requires that we reconcile with the universal truth of impermanence, that all that is born must die. Last, we must relax ideas of ourselves and of the other person. The only thing that matters at this moment is to give this person whom I have been calling my mother the space to die at her own pace. Anything short of that is sure to cause suffering for both her and me.

We tend to make a big deal of death. Watching my mother gently fade away, I am struck by the simple physical nature of the end of life, the same way I felt when my daughters were born, only in reverse. We are born, we live, we die, that's all, and with each transition, we are given to a bunch of physical processes, of entering, being in, and leaving the body. At some point, the body gets worn out and starts shutting down. In the case of Alzheimer's, as with my mom, the end phase stretches over many years, giving loved ones a chance to work with grief and clinging not just once, but numerous times. One thing I have learned from this process is the need to appreciate all that is given at any moment. It is so easy to focus on what no longer is, as opposed to what still is. Before my mother lost the ability to speak a month ago, I did not realize how much it mattered to me that she be able to talk and respond still, even within the limited range of her late-stage Alzheimer's narrative. Now, treasuring the times sitting at her side and feeling her spirit, still flickering, and her breath also, I know soon there will be no life left at all.

Surfing the Grief

We also become freed from our grief and no longer become consumed by it. Each time a new wave comes, we don't get swept away, but instead learn to ride it. Here again is what it feels like inside, using my own example during the month before my mom's passing away.

I could not sleep last night. Grief was compelling me to stay up and investigate. In the darkness, in between breaths, I was able to see grief as the hindrance that it is, an extreme form of aversion to the nature of life itself. My mind wanted to keep on telling stories about my mother and how she used to be, and how I wish she would still be, and how I was not ready to face the final nature of our parting. I noticed how much I was getting lost in those thoughts, and I remembered what to do when faced with a hindrance. You focus on the hindrance itself, not the object. Stepping back one notch, away from thoughts about my mother, I turned my attention to the aversion and I asked myself, what is the thing that keeps it going? Beneath, I found clinging and magical thinking, a deeply seated delusion about life not ending, or ending only on my own terms. And I was able to face the hard truth, of the inevitability of life passing. Later, during dinner with my daughter, I could feel the grief threatening to take over and spoil those precious moments with her. And I realized the foolishness of indulging such a mind state right then. The situation called for no less than appreciating the tenderness between us, and the joy of our good meal together.

Mindfulness is what helps us notice each wave. Wisdom and a deeper understanding of what is make it possible for us to not drown in the thoughts and emotions, so that we can show up for the present moment and all it offers.

Opening the Gifts

One of the benefits of mindfulness practice is the progressive discovery of the many gifts that come from being on the dementia journey. These gifts result from a change of heart and from a different way of viewing oneself, the other person, and the dementia experience.

Dementia Gifts for the Mindful Caregiver

Presence
We discover the best way to engage the person who is living with dementia, which is also the only way to be if we are really wise, for that is the only real moment we have.

Tranquility
By practicing staying in the present, we can learn to let go of ruminations about the past and worries about the future.

Authenticity

We discover the relief of the authentic self, which gets called upon when we relate to a person with dementia.

Love

Dementia forces us to discover true love in the form of love given unconditionally, without any expectation of being loved in return.

Freedom

We are called to free ourselves internally from rigid roles, expectations, patterns of relating, and old scripts.

Gratitude

We become more grateful and learn to savor simple daily pleasures that we may have overlooked before, when our expectations of happiness were higher.

Creativity

We are led to tap into our natural creativity to improvise new roles and find new solutions, in response to constantly changing and unpredictable needs.

Wholeness

Being with the totality of our experience, not pushing anything away, including difficult thoughts and emotions, we realize our natural wholeness.

Humor

It is not all doom and gloom. Mindfulness helps us catch those moments of lightness when the dementia way of being is simply too funny not to laugh.

Wisdom

Dementia forces us to reach down to deeper layers of ourselves, beyond surface thinking, emotional reactivity, and compulsive doing. There we find true wisdom.

Patience

We learn the gift of patience because we have to. Through a process of trial and error, we find that impatience is a dead end that only makes things worse.

Joy

Probably the greatest gift of all is the discovery of the joy that comes when we are fully present to our experience, with our whole being.

INQUIRY:
Discovering Your Own Gifts

Write down all the gifts you have received from caring for a person with dementia. Those gifts may appear in the form of images, words, or feelings. You can also spend a minute on each of the gifts in the list above, and reflect to see whether or not it applies to you. If you are more visually inclined, you might also make a collage out of all your gifts. Realize that this is a dynamic and very personal process.

Practicing Forward

Now is a good time to revisit the main practices you have learned in this book.

Twenty-Five Mindful Care Practices to Remember

1. STOP

2. Awareness of breath

3. Self-compassion break

4. Care partnering

5. Repositioning

6. Enabling decision making

7. Sitting with

8. Mindful walking

9. Mindful walking with

10. Body scan

11. Meeting the need to feel useful

12. Mindfulness of sounds

13. Walking with the four elements

14. Mindful eating

15. Mindfulness of hindrances

16. Loving-kindness

17. Opening the heart door

18. Before meeting

19. Taking in the good

20. Mindfulness of thoughts

21. Aikido communication

22. Mindfulness of feeling

23. Bookend practice

24. Relaxing the self

25. Practicing together (with the person in our care)

Practice Plan

Usually caregivers come away with a list of favorite practices. The number of practices is not so important as the dedication to actually carry on with them. To start your practice plan, list the mindfulness practices that have been most useful to you and ways in which they have helped. Then, write down the things that will help you keep up your mindfulness practice. Also write down obstacles to practice, if any, and how you can overcome them. Finally, write about your main take-away from this book. A downloadable form to help you with this available at http://www.newharbinger.com/31571.

I'd like to close with these words from Olivia Ames Hoblitzelle (2008, 170):

> Remember that caregiving is as hard as anything you've ever done. Whatever happens—and we know all the unpredictable, alarming things that can—the most valuable response is your steady, calm, and caring presence.

Resources

Websites

Mindfulness

Insight Meditation Center: http://www.insightmeditationcenter.org
/books-articles/meditation-instruction/ (good instructions to get
started with mindfulness practice)

Mindfulness-Based Dementia Care (MBDC): Presence Care Project:
http://www.presencecareproject.com (includes free audio files)

Mindfulness-Based Stress Reduction (MBSR): Center for
Mindfulness in Medicine, Health Care, and Society: http://
www.umassmed.edu/cfm

Spirit Rock Meditation Center: http://www.spiritrock.org

UCLA Mindful Awareness Research Center: http://www.marc.ucla
.edu/body.cfm?id=22 (free guided meditations)

Caregiving and Dementia Care

Aging Life Care Association (formerly National Association of
Professional Geriatric Care Managers): http://www.caremanager
.org

Alzheimer's Disease Education and Referral Center (ADEAR):
https://www.nia.nih.gov/alzheimers

Alzheimer's Association Trial Match (connects people with Alzheimer's and their caregivers to current studies): http://www.alz.org/research/clinical_trials/find_clinical_trials_trialmatch.asp

Alzheimer's Association: http://www.alz.org

American Parkinson Disease Association (APDA): http://parkinsons.stanford.edu (great resource for PD with dementia and atypical parkinsonism conditions, including Lewy body dementia)

Association for Frontotemporal Degeneration (AFTD): http://www.theaftd.org

Clinical Trials: https://www.clinicaltrials.gov

Family Caregiver Alliance: https://www.caregiver.org (free home assessments and respite grants)

Lewy Body Dementia Association (LBDA): https://www.lbda.org

Mayo Clinic: http://www.mayoclinic.org/patient-care-and-health-information

National Adult Day Services Association (NADSA): http://www.nadsa.org

National Association of Area Agencies on Aging: http://www.n4a.org

National Elder Law Foundation: http://nelf.org

Neurocern (dementia screening and personalized care resources): http://www.neurocern.com

UCSF Memory and Aging Center: memory.ucsf.edu (most complete resource to learn about the latest dementia science and research, including different types of dementia)

Readings

Hanson, Rick (neuropsychologist), *Buddha's Brain*. New Harbinger Publications, 2009.

Hoblitzelle, Olivia Ames (dementia caregiver), *Ten Thousand Joys and Ten Thousand Sorrows*. Penguin, 2008.

Kabat-Zinn, Jon (founder of MBSR), *Full Catastrophe Living: Using the Wisdom of Your Body and Mind to Face Stress, Pain, and Illness*. Bantam Dell, 1990.

Neff, Kristin (researcher), *Self-Compassion*. HarperCollins, 2011.

Pearce, Nancy (geriatric social worker), *Inside Alzheimer's*. Forrason Press, 2007.

Power, Allen (geriatrician), *Dementia Beyond Drugs: Changing the Culture of Care*. Health Professions Press, 2010.

References

Alzheimer's Association. *2015 Alzheimer's Disease Facts and Figures.* Chicago.

Behrman, S., L. Chouliaras, and K. Ebmeier. 2014. "Considering the Senses in the Diagnosis and Management of Dementia." *Maturitas* 77: 305–10.

Boss, P. 1999. *Ambiguous Loss: Learning to Live with Unresolved Grief.* Cambridge: Harvard University Press.

Bryden, C. 2005. *Dancing with Dementia: My Story of Living Positively with Dementia.* London: Jessica Kingsley Publishers.

Burns, D. 1989. *The Feeling Good Handbook: Using the New Mood Therapy in Everyday Life.* New York: W. Morrow.

Collier, L. 2014. *Living Sensationally with Dementia—Understanding How We Use Our Senses.* http://rompa.com/media/free-resources/sensory-processing-in-dementia-alzheimers-show-2014.pdf.

Denison, R. 2010. Recorded talk during Women's Retreat at Dhamma Dena Retreat Center, fall 2010.

Doka, K. 2010. "Grief, Multiple Loss, and Dementia." *Bereavement Care* 29: 15–20.

Epel, E., E. Blackburn, J. Lin, F. Dhabhar, N. Adler, J. Morrow, and R. Cawthon. 2004. "Accelerated Telomere Shortening in Response to Life Stress." *Proceedings of the National Academy of Sciences of the United States of America* 101: 17312–5.

Epel, E., J. Daubenmier, J. Moskowitz, S. Folkman, and E. Blackburn. 2009. "Can Meditation Slow Rate of Cellular Aging? Cognitive Stress, Mindfulness, and Telomeres." *Annals of the New York Academy of Sciences* 1172: 34–53.

Fogg, BJ. 2011. *Tiny Habits.* http://tinyhabits.com/.

Frank, J. 2008. "Evidence for Grief as the Major Barrier Faced by Alzheimer Caregivers: A Qualitative Analysis." *American Journal of Alzheimer's Disease and Other Dementias* 22: 241–53.

Gordon, S. 2010. "Sitting Docs Have Happier Patients." *U.S. News and World Report:* http://health.usnews.com/health-news/managing-your -healthcare/healthcare/articles/2010/04/07/sitting-docs-have -happier-patients.

Hanh, Thich Nhat. *Transforming Anger.* YouTube video, 5:00. Posted by "Ratanayano Bhikkhu," January 6, 2015. https://www.youtube.com /watch?v=UPVr6w_P67c.

Hanson, R. 2009. *Buddha's Brain.* Oakland: New Harbinger Publications.

Hanson, R. 2010. "Confronting the Negativity Bias." http://www.rick hanson.net/your-wise-brain/how-your-brain-makes-you-easily -intimidated.

Hoblitzelle, O. 2008. *Ten Thousand Joys and Ten Thousand Sorrows.* New York: Penguin.

Kabat-Zinn, J. 1994. *Wherever You Go, There You Are: Mindfulness Meditation in Everyday Life.* New York: Hyperion.

Khema, A. 1987. *Being Nobody, Going Nowhere: Meditations on the Buddhist Path.* Somerville, MA: Wisdom Publications.

Killingsworth, M., and D. Gilbert. 2010. "A Wandering Mind Is an Unhappy Mind." *Science* 330: 932.

Lyubomirsky, S., K. Sheldon, and D. Schkade. 2005. "Pursuing Happiness: The Architecture of Sustainable Change." *Review of General Psychology* 9: 111–131.

Neff, K. 2015. Self-Compassion website: http://self-compassion.org.

Power, A. 2010. *Dementia Beyond Drugs: Changing the Culture of Care.* Baltimore: Health Professions Press.

Scientific Report of the 2015 Dietary Guidelines Advisory Committee (Advisory Report) to the Secretaries of the U.S. Department of Health and Human Services (HHS) and the U.S. Department of Agriculture (USDA). http:// health.gov/dietaryguidelines/2015-scientific-report.

Selver, C. 2007. "Every Moment Is a Moment of Learning." Recorded video, Sensory Awareness Foundation.

Smith, M., and K. Buckwalter. 2006. *Back to the A-B-C's: Understanding and Responding to Behavioral Symptoms in Dementia.* Cedar Rapids, IA: John A. Hartford Center of Geriatric Nursing Excellence, College of Nursing, University of Iowa.

Spitzer, R., J. Williams, K. Kroenke et al. 1999. "Patient Health Questionnaire–9" (PHQ-9). Pfizer Inc.

Vasilopoulos, H. 2010. *Sensory Impairments Across the Life Span.* http:// www.thedementiaspecialist.com/si_across_lifespan6hr.pdf.

Verity, J. 2015. *Spark of Life 5 Core Emotional Needs.* http://www.dementia careaustralia.com/index.php?option=com_content&task=view&id =731&Itemid=81.

Marguerite Manteau Rao, LCSW, is a licensed clinical social worker specializing in bringing new, innovative solutions to the field of dementia care. She is CEO of the Presence Care Project and was founder of the MindfulnessBased Dementia Care program at the Osher Center for Integrative Medicine at the University of California, San Francisco. She is also cofounder of Neurocern, a software company aimed at empowering dementia caregivers with neuroscience-based, person-centered care solutions. Manteau-Rao is also a contributor to *The Huffington Post*.

Foreword writer **Kevin Barrows, MD**, is clinical professor of family and community medicine at the School of Medicine at the University of California, San Francisco. He is founder and director of mindfulness programs at the Osher Center for Integrative Medicine, where he helps patients cope with the stress of everyday life and illness.

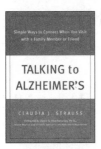
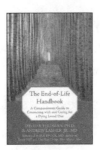
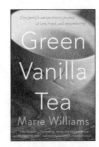
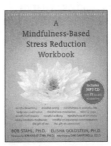
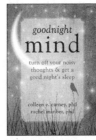 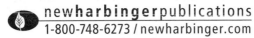

Register your **new harbinger** titles for additional benefits!

When you register your **new harbinger** title—purchased in any format, from any source—you get access to benefits like the following:

- Downloadable accessories like printable worksheets and extra content

- Instructional videos and audio files

- Information about updates, corrections, and new editions

Not every title has accessories, but we're adding new material all the time.

Access free accessories in 3 easy steps:

1. Sign in at NewHarbinger.com (or **register** to create an account).

2. Click on **register a book**. Search for your title and click the **register** button when it appears.

3. Click on the **book cover or title** to go to its details page. Click on **accessories** to view and access files.

That's all there is to it!

If you need help, visit:

NewHarbinger.com/accessories

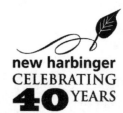

new harbinger
CELEBRATING
40 YEARS